AORTO-CORONARY BYPASS SURGERY

AORTO-CORONARY BYPASS SURGERY

BEERT BUIS, M. D.

Department of Cardiology, Leiden University Hospital

H. E. STENFERT KROESE B.V. – LEIDEN 1974

ISBN 978-90-207-0474-7   ISBN 978-94-011-9633-8 (eBook)
DOI 10.1007/978-94-011-9633-8

CONTENTS

CHAPTER 1

INTRODUCTION

Summary

A comprehensive review is given of the literature, and the advantages
and disadvantages of the bypass operation are discussed in detail.

Of all surgical interventions aiming at revascularisation of the myocardium the aorto-coronary bypass operation is the one which indoubtedly has earned its place in cardiac surgery.

The most suitable candidates for this operation are those with a normal left ventricular angiogram and a good peripheral vascular pattern. Even in these people the question still remains whether the vein can stay patent for many years; moreover what happens to the proximal coronary arteries is as yet uncertain.

In the case of poorly contracting ventricles little good is to be expected from the by-pass operation. Possible, anastomosis of the internal mammary artery with a stenotic coronary artery merits preference over a venous bypass. To demonstrate the ultimate influence of this type of surgical intervention on life expectance and on a secondary prevention of angina pectoris and myocardial infarction, Chalmers (1972) and Spodick (1971) favour follow-up studies of patients who are divided at random into a surgical and a non-surgical group.

1.1. OBJECT

The object of this investigation is to establish on basis of the results and complications of saphenous vein bypass grafting (briefly termed bypass surgery):
– reliable indications for this operation;
– to provide the surgeon with a guide to the choice of surgical technique.

1.2. LITERATURE

1.2.1. Surgical methods

The first attempt to relieve anginous complaints by means of surgery was made many decades ago.

In 1899 François Frank suggested severing the nerve fibres of the heart thus elimin-
ating the pain. It was not until 1920, however, that this method was applied by Jonnesco.
In contrast to this operation which did not influence the supply of blood to the myocardium, many operations have been described during the last thirty years, which were
designed for precisely this purpose.

The blood supply to the myocardium can be increased in two ways:

– indirectly;
– directly.

An indirect method is understood to be an operation on the muscle tissue of the heart,
whereas the direct method implies an operation on the coronary arteries.

An example of indirect surgery is the approach made by Beck who in 1935 described
an operation involving extirpation of the pericardium, the aim being to promote the
growth of new vessels to the myocardium.

Later a number of modifications were added. Some surgeons e.g. attached the greater
omentum to the pericardium and there were others who insufflated talcum into the
pericardium (Thompson, 1949), all hoping to promote the growth of new vessels to the
pericardium and the myocardium. Of the indirect methods the one applied mostly is that
according to Vineberg (1962). He made a tunnel into the myocardium and laid in it an
internal mammary artery which had been previously detached from the surrounding
tissue.

At first the operations were performed only on animals and then, in 1950, the technique
was used on humans for the first time. In 1954, twelve patients in the U.S.A. were
operated on according to this method. A report of the American College of Chest Surgeons (May) published in 1968 contained a review of 3787 patients who had undergone
such an operation.

Mortality as a result of the operation was 5.9% when one internal mammary artery was
implanted and rose to 7.5% when both mammary arteries were brought to the myocardium.

Vineberg (1962) himself, reports a lower figure, viz. 2.9%. Post-operative roentgenology
with injection of contrast medium showed that 40% of the implanted arteries were still
functioning after ten months. In 20% of the patients a connection had even formed between the internal mammary artery and the left coronary artery.

The performance and assessment of revascularisation operations received a great
stimulus in 1959 when Mason Sones described selective coronary arteriography. The
operation introduced by Vineberg was employed on a large scale, particularly in the
U.S.A. Led by the surgeons Effler (1971) and Favaloro (1968), the Cleveland Group
operated on many patients.

In spite of the fact that the complaints diminished postoperatively, doubts soon arose.
An investigation by Langston showed that the complaints were clearly less in a number

of patients while both mammary arteries were not functioning. Objective improvement in the sense of increased toleration of effort, improved left ventricle function and positively improved blood supply to the myocardium, could never be demonstrated. Thus, with the aid of an electromagnetic flowmeter Dart (1970) found that the mean blood flow through the implanted vessel was 8 ml/min. Since the normal blood flow through the coronary arteries is 50-120 ml/min./100 g heart muscle tissue, it cannot be assumed that such a small quantity as 8 ml/min. really contributes to an improved blood supply to the myocardium.

Taylor (1967) demonstrated that the lactate production of the myocardium diminished after implantation of one or both internal mammary arteries. This might indicate a reduction of the ischaemia in the heart muscle, but it could also be indicative of the preoperative ischaemic region being scarred, as it is known that this would cease production of lactate, even under load. Gradually other ways of improving the supply of blood to the heart muscle were sought.

Senning (1961) opened the coronary artery over the stenosed region and after the lumen had been cleared the defect was closed with a pericardial patch. This operation was associated with a high mortality and, moreover, the results were unsatisfactory, giving a poor patency rate.

The same was experienced with direct endarterectomy (Effler, 1964). It is true that reasonable results were obtained for the right coronary artery, but for the left coronary artery the mortality was high (50%).

It was already known from peripheral vascular surgery (Baddely, 1970; Caldwell, 1968; Darling, 1967) that when a vein is placed between the proximal and distal parts of an artery, the vein may remain patent for quite a long time provided the run-off is good.

Factors such as length of the vein, hypertension or diabetes seem to be of minor importance for a good result.

In analogy to this Favaloro (1967) replaced the stenosed part of a coronary artery by a piece of vein and in this way tried to improve the blood supply to the distal coronary artery. There were two major objections:

– the operation was associated with high mortality;
– the patency rate was low.

As early as 1954 Murray described the possibility of joining an artery to a coronary artery; in 1966 (Effler, 1971) Kahn was the first to place a vein between the aorta and a coronary artery in a human being. This technique was called: Saphenous Vein Bypass Grafting – provided, of course, that a saphenous vein was used. Two great clinics in the U.S.A. were among the first to introduce saphenous vein bypass grafting. Those concerned were Effler (1971) and Favaloro (1971) in Cleveland and Johnson (1969, 1970) in Milwaukee.

The theoretical background of this operation in which the anastomosis of the aorta with the coronary artery is made distally of the stenosed region is based on two facts:

- a vein placed between two arteries can remain open for years;
- in most cases of coronary sclerosis the stenosis is located in the proximal part of the vessel, while the distal wall of the vessel is normal.

Blumgart (1940) and James (1961) found by autopsy that the changes were located predominantly in the proximal part of the coronary vessels. These findings have been confirmed again by Green (1970), who anastomosed the internal mammary artery with a coronary artery. He found in almost all patients with a serious stenosis in the anterior descending branch of the left coronary artery, at the level of 1.0 mm a patent vessel.

1.2.2. Indications for saphenous vein bypass grafting

Johnson (1969-70), Effler (1971) and Favaloro (1969-70) give five prerequisites for this operation:

   I. The patients must be suffering from anginous complaints;
  II. The stenoses in the coronary arteries should fill at least 75% of the lumen;
 III. The bypassed coronary artery should supply a substantial part of the myocardium with blood;
  IV. The muscle of the left ventricle should not be damaged too much;
   V. The diameter of the vessel should be large enough to permit distal anastomosis.

I. It is difficult to express the patient's symptoms in terms of numbers or make correlations between subjective symptoms and objective signs such as exercise ECG since they are not reported as indications for the bypass operation. An exception is made for patients with a serious stenosis of the main trunk of the left coronary artery. This defect is said to be accompanied by a high mortality, even in patients who have few complaints (Cohn, 1971).

II. The stenosis in the coronary artery should fill about 70-75% of the lumen. This condition is based on the finding by Johnson who, in the course of performing operations, found no gradient over the stenosis if it did not fill at least 70% of the lumen. From this he concluded that the flow decreased only when a very severe stenosis was present.

Furuse (1972) found in animal experiments that the total flow through a bypass and a coronary artery is determined by the distal run-off. When a vein is introduced between the aorta and a coronary artery and the flow of blood through the original coronary artery is artificially reduced by 10% by applying a constriction, the 10 per cent will immediately be taken over by the venous bypass. Even if the coronary artery is not stenosed, it is possible that more than 50% of the total quantity of blood passing through the relevant coronary artery prior to the venous bypass being established will now pass through the vein. As a consequence the proximal stenosis can become occluded with sludge owing to the small flow.

III. The coronary artery which is to be anastomosed with a vein should supply a substantial part of the myocardium with blood, otherwise the flow through the vein will be too small which may lead to occlusion.

IV. The myocardium should not be seriously damaged. In Effler's (1971) view there is no point in bringing blood to a scar. In this connection it should be noted that sometimes it is difficult to make a distinction between ischaemic regions and regions consisting solely of scar tissue (Johnson, 1970).

V. Distal of the stenosis the lumen of the coronary artery should be about 2 mm in diameter. It has been found in practice that a satisfactory anastomosis can be applied to such a vessel. It is, of course, possible to connect a vessel to smaller vessels, but there is great risk that a vein connected in this way will become occluded. Here the coronary angiographic examination is of great value, since it has been found that the estimated diameter established during the operation is in good agreement with the diameter estimated via coronary angiography. This does not apply to those cases where the coronary artery fills via collaterals; it is then often wider in reality than supposed from the angiogram.

1.2.3. Contra-indications for bypass procedure

Effler (1971) and Favaloro (1971) consider that there is no point in giving a patient a bypass if the wall of the left ventricle gives evidence of scarcely any movement in the angiogram. Johnson (1970) regards acute myocardial infarction as the only contra-indication. A number of authors voice some objections to bypass surgery. These have been well stated by Friedberg (1972) and may be summarised as follows:

- In 10% of patients who have undergone bypass surgery, the electrocardiogram shows an infarct pattern (Q or QS) immediately after operation.
- The subtotal stenosis in the proximal coronary artery can become total as result of the bypass operation (Bourassa, 1972).
- In the course of time, changes can occur in the venous walls, which may lead to stenosis or even total occlusion (Johnson, 1970).
- The operation can result in myocardial lesion.
- The risk of (re-)infarction in, and the survival period of, patients who have undergone this operation are insufficiently known.

1.2.4. Surgical technique

1.2.4.1. Surgical technique in venous bypass procedure
It is known from surgery of the peripheral vessels (Kishiskian and Furuse, 1972) that to ensure a good anastomosis between two vessels, the difference in calibre should be as small as possible. If there is a serious luminal disproportion between graft and recipient artery turbulences can occur and promote occlusion by sludging. At the beginning of by-pass surgery the great saphenous vein was taken from the thigh. As this vein was too large, in many cases, it was decided to take veins from the lower leg. In order to prevent damage to the intima it is necessary that great care be exercised in detaching the vein from the surrounding tissue. Flushing the vein with a physiological saline solution is not advised. The valves may not be removed (risk of lesion to intima) and, in order not to obstruct the flow, the vein is implanted in reverse direction, so that the direction of blood flow in the vein is the same as it was during the time when the vessel was a leg vein. Small venules should be tied off as short as possible so that no bulges are left in the veins (fig. 1). The anastomosis is performed with the aid of extra-corporeal circulation.

If possible, the aorta is not clamped off; if this is unavoidable, however, it should be for as short a time as possible.

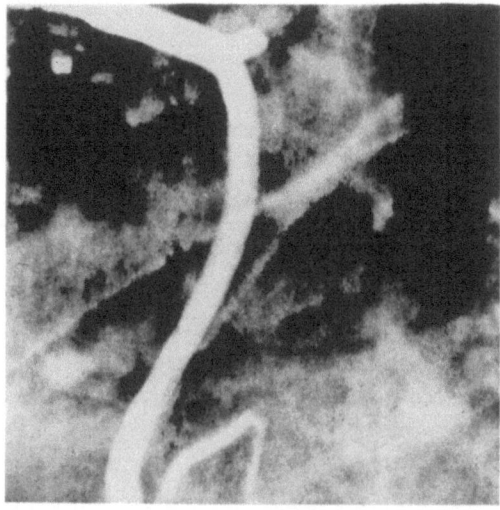

Fig. 1. Saphenous vein graft to left anterior descending in left anterior oblique projection. Note pouch in the graft.

After a few weeks or months a vein will shrink somewhat, becoming shorter. As a result the anastomosed parts may be stretched so tightly that they close. This will occur particularly with a vein interposed between the aorta and the left coronary artery. The vein should therefore be routed in a wide curve.

Effler et al. (1971), Favaloro (1971) and Reul (1971-72) give no special guidance to pre-operative preparation except for advising that medication with beta-blockers be stopped prior to the operation.

Johnson (1970) advises complete digitalisation, potassium supplementation and the blood volume at full level; he prefers to operate with a high haematocrit value.

Adam (1970) sees no point in administering heparine and cumarine in the post-operative phase, but does give acetosal to prevent clotting of the blood platelets and with it occlusion of the anastomosed parts due to sludge formation.

1.2.4.2. Surgical technique of endarterectomy

Hahn (1972) believes that an endarterectomy is of value in 90% of venous bypasses to the right coronary artery. When endarterectomy is performed, the atheromatous matter is removed – after the vessel has been opened – either manually or with carbon dioxide. In cases in which a lumen can scarcely be seen in the coronary angiogram, venous bypasses can still be made by employing this technique. To some extent this view is contested by Danielson who considers that the patency rate of the veins is lower after an endarterectomy of the recipient coronary artery has been performed than if endarterectomy is omitted.

In nine of ten patients who had undergone gas endarterectomy Benchimol (1972) observed post-operative infarction.

Kaplitt (1971) agrees with Hahn that a useful purpose is served by performing endarterectomy. He found that when this method is employed in cadavers, even the smallest branches can still be emptied of the atheromatous matter.

1.2.4.3. Surgical technique when use is made of the internal mammary artery

In 1967 Kolessov described the possibility of anastomosing the internal mammary artery directly with the coronary vessel.

The technique has been promoted by Green who has achieved many successes with it. The advantages over a venous graft are:
- Anastomosis between two arteries is more physiological in character.
- The diameter of the internal mammary artery and that of the average coronary artery correspond better.
- Only one anastomosis is needed instead of two.
- If the anastomosis has been well performed the patency rate after one year is 97%, even in those cases where a low flow is found.
- After one year no changes have been observed in the wall of the internal mammary artery.

The disadvantages of using the internal mammary artery as compared with venous grafts are:

- The surgical technique is somewhat more difficult and the surgeon requires optical enlargement for the small vessels which have a diameter of 1 to 1½ mm.
- The average flow through an internal mammary artery is lower than through an average venous bypass.
- Only two arteries are present. This could be offset by using the splenic artery (Edwards, 1972).

The fact that an internal mammary artery continues to function well, even when the flow of blood through the artery is low, seems to be a particularly strong argument in those cases where it is technically possible to use an artery instead of a vein (Green, 1970; Johnson, 1970).

1.2.5. Results and complications of bypass procedure

1.2.5.1. Mortality and (re-)infarction
There is a close relation between the surgical risk and the left ventricular function. Many authors determine the function from the left ventricular angiogram. If the wall moves slightly or not at all during systole, one speaks of hypo- or akinesia respectively. This dysfunction can be diffuse as well as local. The more infarcts a patient has had, the greater the risk of the bypass operation having a high mortality. The correlation between the left ventricular angiogram and the number of infarcts experienced is good (Johnson). In the early stages of bypass surgery Johnson (1969) had an operative mortality of 37% in patients with serious myocardial defects. Later the incidence could be reduced to 8%.

In 1971 Effler, for a normal or slightly aberrant left ventricular angiogram, reported operative mortality incidences of 2.5%, 3.5% and 4.7% respectively for single, double and triple saphenous vein bypass grafting.

Yatteau observed a rise in operational mortality when the ejection fraction (percentage of the diastolic volume that is ejected in systole) was 25% or less.

Chalmers (1972) made a literature survey covering twenty-eight publications on bypass surgery and he found that institutions in which many operations were performed had a lower mortality. In the case of two-hundred or more operations per year, the average mortality was 4.5% (3.484 patients). This figure relates to six institutions. Those in which one to two-hundred operations are performed per year have a mortality of 9% (1.255 patients in eight institutions). In the remaining fourteen, having less than one-hundred operations per year, mortality ranged from 0 to 26.5% (512 patients).

Factors such as diabetes, hypertension and hypercholesterolemia do not appear to have any great significance for the direct operative mortality (Kong, 1971). Factors that can increase the risk, however, are accompanying mitral insufficiency, signs of decompensation or of an end-diastolic pressure higher than 25 mm Hg in the left ventricle (Cooley, 1972).

Some of the larger centres published figures on the (re-)infarction and the mortality incidence when patients have left the hospital after the operation.

Sheldon (1972) studied one-thousand patients who had been operated on in the period 1967-70. Data on 97.2% of these patients were available over a follow-up period of 22-60 months. Including the operative mortality of 4% in his calculation, he found that 79.4% of these patients were still alive after five years. According to the same author, of a similar group of patients who had not been operated on, 65.8% were still alive after five years.

MacRaven (1972) found that in a follow-up period of six months the mortality was 1% if the left ventricle contracted normally. This figure could rise to 6% for a poorly contracting ventricle.

There are also some publications on the life expectancy of patients in relation to the anatomic aberrations. Thus Lichtlen (1972) found in two-hundred and thirty-one patients followed up during a period of up to thirty-two months that the mortality was 10% if one coronary vessel was subject to serious atherosclerotic narrowing. If three vessels were affected this figures rose to 34%.

Moberg (1972) reported that when three vessels were affected a mortality of 70% occurred in the period from seven to nine years.

Bruschke (1973) also observed an increase in mortality when more than one vessel was affected.

1.2.5.2. Electrocardiographic changes

In about 10% of the patients who had been operated on, the ECG showed directly post-operative signs of myocardial infarction (Hultgren, 1971; Friedberg, 1972; Greenberg, 1971; Reul, 1971). These ECG findings are not related solely to the functioning of the venous bypass, since the Q-waves are observed directly after the operation, in both occluded and patent venous bypasses.

Aldridge (1971) drew attention to the influence which patent bypass can exercise on the proximal coronary artery. The flow through the stenosed region can decrease and the stenosis – which was formerly sub-total – can become total after the operation. Side-branches of the proximal part can become sludged in this way with the result that in-farction might occur.

Bourassa (1972) saw in 20% of the cases of the vein being closed off, that the proximal sub-total stenosis had become total. If the vein was still patent then the proximal coronary artery was found to be closed in 30% of the cases.

1.2.5.3. Patency rate

A number of factors can be responsible for the bypass sludging up:

– Biological influences (e.g. fibroplasia and thrombosis).
– Physiological influences (e.g. distal run-off and progression of the disease).
– Trauma (e.g. suturing technique and construction at the level of the side-branches).

In this connection Vlodaver (1971) and Edwards (1971) have described two processes which can occur in an anstomosed vein, viz.:

– Thrombosis.
  This is probably ascribable to a sluggish blood flow. This can be prevented by making the anastomosis wide, while no constrictions may be made in the vein and the recipient coronary artery. The peripheral vascular bed should be large enough to guarantee a good distal run-off.
– Fibrous proliferation of the intima.
  Fibroblasts and acid mucopolysaccharides occur in the intima and are responsible for these changes. It would be incorrect to term this process arterialisation, since an artery has a thicker media than a vein and the proliferation occurs in the intima.

Johnson (1970) found these changes already present in some veins prior to implantation. Exactly how these changes occur is not known; they might possibly be the result of a water-hammer effect of the systolic pressure. It should be regarded mainly as being that the total quantity of blood flowing through the vein is small. It is remarkable that arteriosclerotic changes in the veins are hardly ever observed.

The percentage of veins which are stated as being closed immediately after the operation is as follows. In 1972 Walker reported early occlusion in 12% of cases. Effler and Favaloro give about the same figures. Many authors ascribe this early occlusion to an imperfect operation technique. Walker (1971) related the flow measured during the operation to the post-operative patency. The early patency rate with an average flow of 41 ml/min. or more was 90%. If on the other hand the flow was less than 40 ml/min. then the patency rate was 75%.

Sheldon (1972) reported that 83.7% of the veins were still patent after twenty-five months. Walker (1972) noted late occlusion in 13% of the veins. If the veins are patent immediately after operation, the foremost factor for late occlusion appears to be the fibrous intima hyperplasia, unless small irregularities and bulges are already present immediately following operation (figs. 1 and 2); these can give rise to later occlusion (Bourassa).

Johnson and Bourassa (1970-72) have noted a diminution of diameter in the vein. The latter author found that the diminution occurs in the first year after the operation;

in a follow-up check three years after the operation he observed no further decrease in diameter.

Walker (1971) found that the late patency rate was 46% when the average flow measured during operation was 40 ml/min. or lower.

Green (1970) gave figures concerning one-hundred and fifty-two patients with a follow-up period of at least six months. A venous graft was made in eighty-four patients; forty-three were given a double vein graft. In all of them the internal mammary artery was anastomosed with a coronary artery. Of the seventy patients who were catheterised afterwards, it was found that the internal mammary artery was occluded in 3%; occlusion rates of 30% were found for the veins.

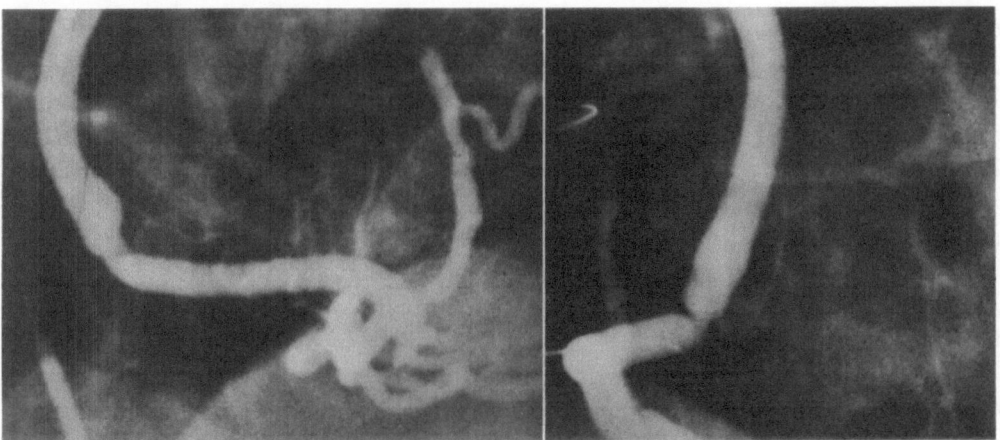

Fig. 2. Saphenous vein graft to right coronary artery. Direct post-operative localized stenosis.
Left: right anterior oblique projection.
Right: left anterior oblique projection.

1.2.5.4. Non-cardial complications

Compared with other surgical operations which are performed with the aid of extra-corporeal circulation, the complications were not greater. Reul (1972) in a review of one-thousand and twenty-two patients reported serious neurological changes in 1% of the cases and grave respiratory complications in 2%.

1.2.5.5. Complaints and validity

All the great institutions report that six months to one year after the operation no, or much fewer, complaints were present in 85% of the patients.

Friedberg (1972) and Chalmers (1972) point out that disappearance of the complaints need not necessarily be the result of a properly functioning bypass.

Dimond and co-workers (1960) found that an improvement was experienced in 65% of the patients who had undergone a sham operation.

The worst results were seen by Reul (1971-72) and Cooley (1972) in patients who had suffered a decompensation. In agreement with this, MacRaven (1972) observed the least improvement in patients who had had disturbed left ventricular function.

A clear improvement in validity as assessed in accordance with the criteria of the New York Heart Association was found by Morris (1972).

Matlof (1972) carried out pre- and post-operative examinations in seventy-one patients. For the group of patients, who had improved the ratio of patent veins to the total number of those implanted was 77:89; in contrast, the ratio for the non-improved group was 12:25.

1.2.5.6. *Ergometric examination and left ventricular function*
During effort the oxygen requirement of the myocardium will increase. If the possibilities for this are inadequate (coronary sclerosis) the following phenomena can occur: pain, electrocardiographic changes, rise in end-diastolic pressure of the left ventricle and diminished contractility. When a bypass has improved the supply of blood to the myocardium, it can be expected that the above phenomena will be absent or will occur only at a higher load.

Bartel (1972) found that those patients whose symptoms had diminished had a better capacity for effort, and that exercise ECG abnormalities present prior to operation disappeared post-operatively.

After a successful operation Johnson (1970) and Campeau (1971) found a normal value for the end-diastolic pressure of the left ventricle for a load which pre-operatively had caused a raised end-diastolic pressure in the left ventricle.

Miller (1972) and Manly (1970) likewise observed improved capacity for effort in the case of a bypass that had remained patent; this was attained by a higher value of the product of the heart rate and systolic blood pressure (H.R. $\times$ B.P.s). For the individual patient this product is a good yardstick for the oxygen consumption of the myocardium. The left ventricular function as assessed from the contractions shown on the angiogram can improve under the influence of a good bypass (Johnson, 1970; Bourassa, 1972; Kline, 1972).

In contrast, however, Dorcahk (1971) sometimes observed the occurrence of an abnormal left ventricular angiogram with a patent bypass.

CHAPTER 2

ROUTINE CLINICAL INVESTIGATION

Summary

A classification into 5 groups of patients is given, according to contraction patterns on the angiogram and to accompanying cardiac abnormalities. The Judkin's method was employed for the coronary angiograms. All patients were catheterised pre-operatively, 2 weeks post-operatively and 12 months post-operatively. In 3 patients, however, no catheterisation was performed post-operatively. Prior to operation and 6 months after surgery the patients were subjected to a maximal exercise-test on the bicycle-ergometer. Diameters of coronary arteries as well as of vein grafts were measured on 70 mm fluorographs with the aid of a microdensitometer. Coronary blood flow was measured during operation.

2.1. PATIENTS

All patients included in this study were referred to the Department of Cardiology and were operated on in the Thoracic Surgical Department of the University Hospital, Leiden. During the period from April 1970 to June 1973, one-hundred and three operations were performed on one-hundred patients. In addition to a bypass operation, a number of patients underwent other surgical intervention, e.g. implantation of a valve prosthesis and/or ventricular aneurysmectomy.

As high operative mortality can be expected with impaired left ventricular contractility patients were classified into five groups on the basis of findings on the left ventricular angiogram:

group 1: normal contraction pattern of left ventricular wall;
group 2: slightly abnormal contraction pattern (fig. 3);
group 3: clearly abnormal contraction pattern;
group 4: aneurysm of the left ventricle (fig. 4);
group 5: patients with an accompanying cardiac abnormality, not as a result of coronary sclerosis.

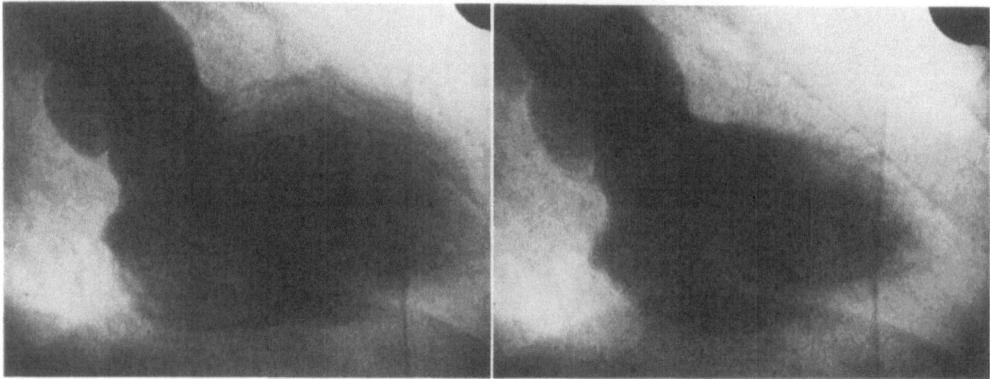

Fig. 3. Left ventricle in right anterior oblique projection, decreased movements of the inferior wall.
Left: diastolic phase.
Right: systolic phase.

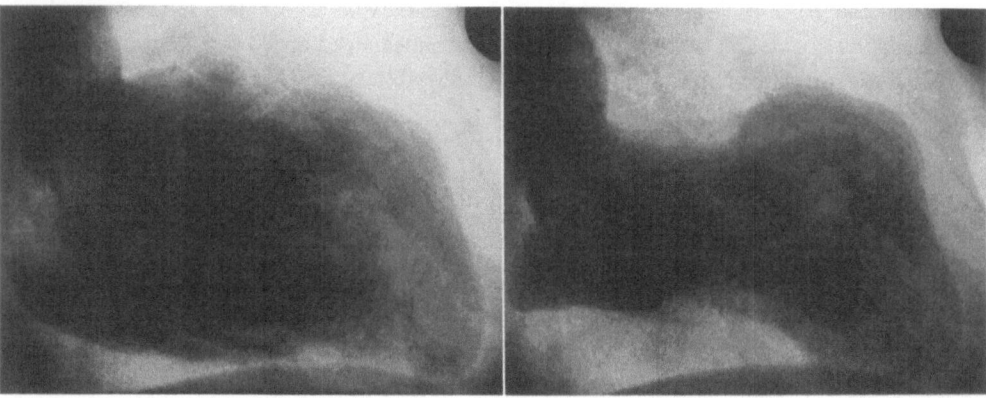

Fig. 4. Left ventricle in right anterior oblique projection, aneurysm around the apex.
Left: diastolic phase.
Right: systolic phase.

Table 1 lists the numbers of patients in each group, age at the time of the operation and sex. The mean age in the five groups was 48, 52, 51, 53 and 50 respectively. The youngest patient was 20, the oldest 66. Of the one-hundred patients, ninety-three were men and seven were women. Group 5 comprised four patients, three of whom had an aortic stenosis and aortic insufficiency; the fourth patient had an ostium stenosis of both coronary arteries as result of syphilitic aortitis.

Table 1. 100 patients with a bypass operation. LV = left ventricle.

LV_Angio	Group	Pts.Nr.	Sex Male	Sex Female	Age years Mean	Age years Range	Direct operative mort. Pts.Nr.	Direct operative mort. Percentage
N	I	47	45	2	48	20_61	3	6.25[x]
+	II	20	18	2	52	43_62	2	10.0
++	III	12	12	-	51	43_61	2	15.3[x]
Aneurysm	IV	17	16	1	53	35_66	2	11.7
Miscella_neous	V	4	2	2	50	43_53	1	20[x]
Total	I_V	100	93	7	50	20_66	10	9.7

N=normal LVangio
+=slightly abnormal LVangio
++=distinct abnormal LVangio

x in each group one patient operated twice

2.2. EXAMINATION METHODS

2.2.1. History and validity

In addition to an extensive history taking, the validity was estimated according to criteria as laid down by the New York Heart Association. Roughly these criteria are defined as follows:

validity 1: no symptoms;
validity 2: symptoms only during heavy physical effort;
validity 3: symptoms during light physical effort;
validity 4: symptoms at rest.

2.2.2. Physical examination, electrocardiogram and X-ray examination of the thorax

The general physical examination was performed in the usual way. A twelve-lead electrocardiogram was recorded on a number of occasions for each patient, and so were röntgenograms of the chest.

2.2.3. Laboratory tests

The serum cholesterol in each patient was determined in addition to the customary tests such as haemoglobine, sedimentation rate, liver, kidney and lung functions.

2.2.4. Exercise electrocardiogram

The work-load was given by means of a bicycle-ergometer, the load being progressively increased with 10 watts each minute. Initially all standard leads were recorded alternately with six precordial leads. In the later phase of the project the standard leads and lead V_5 were assumed to be adequate.

The bicycle test was discontinued if:

1. symptoms of angina became severe;
2. three or more ventricular extra-systoles occurred in succession;
3. the systolic blood pressure dropped during the exercise test;
4. the patient had to give up owing to general fatigue or pain in the legs.

The occurrence of moderate angina with or without ischaemic S-T, T-changes in the electrocardiogram, was not by themselves a reason for stopping the ergometry test. The ECG was recorded before, during and up until fifteen minutes after the test, and the blood pressure was measured with a cuff and the Korotkov sounds and recorded at regular intervals.

2.2.5. Heart catheterisation (see also Appendix, p. 75)

All patients were catheterised using the Seldinger technique, and coronary arteriography was performed as described by Judkins (1968). As a rule patients were not given premedication, except in some cases where a sedative was administered. Anticoagulant dosage was adjusted in such a way that the thrombotest value was one-hundred seconds or shorter, the average normal value being forty-five seconds.

Immediately after insertion of the catheter patients were given 75 mg heparine intra-arterially. Pressures in the left ventricle and the aorta were measured using Statham pressure-transducers and recorded on an eight-channel Hellige photographic writer. End-diastolic pressure was taken to occur at the point where the left ventricular pressure curve rises steeply. If this point could not be clearly identified, the pressure measured 0.05 seconds after onset of QRS was taken as the end-diastolic pressure. The contrast medium used for coronary arteriography and for left ventricular angiography was Isopaque Coronar which contains 370 mg iodine per ml. Prior to injection of the contrast medium, the patient was given $\frac{1}{2}$ mg atropine sulphate intra-arterially and nitroglycerin sublingually. The latter was adjusted to the normal dosage for the relevant patient. The patients were rotated along their longitudinal axes in a cradle, so that left and right oblique studies could be made of the right and left coronary arteries. The X-ray images were recorded with a 35 mm Arriflex camera; in many cases exposures were also made with a 70 mm rapid-sequence camera (figs. 5, 6, 7, 44). Left ventricular angiograms were as a routine procedure made in the right anterior oblique position, unless it was suspected

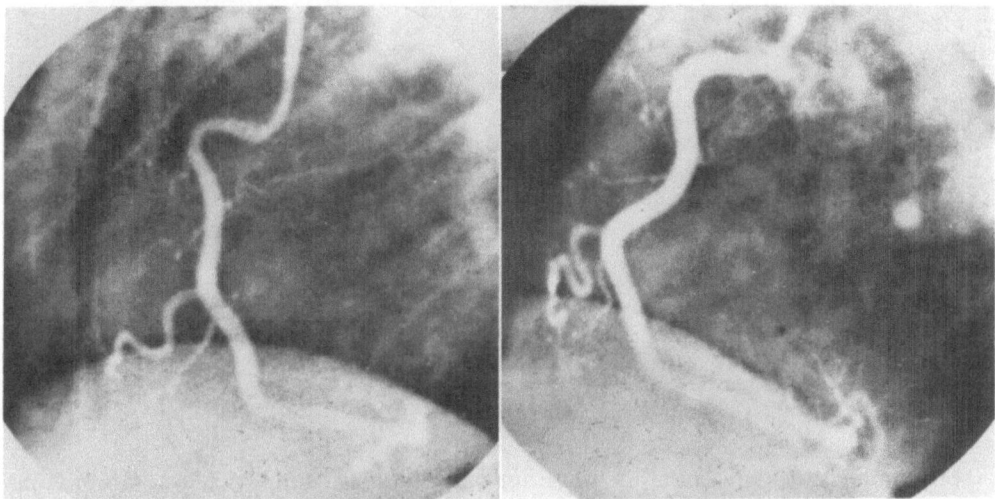

Fig. 5. Right coronary artery in left anterior oblique projection, influence of nitroglycerine.
Left: spasm in the proximal part of the artery.
Right: normal aspects of the artery after administration of nitroglycerine sublingually.

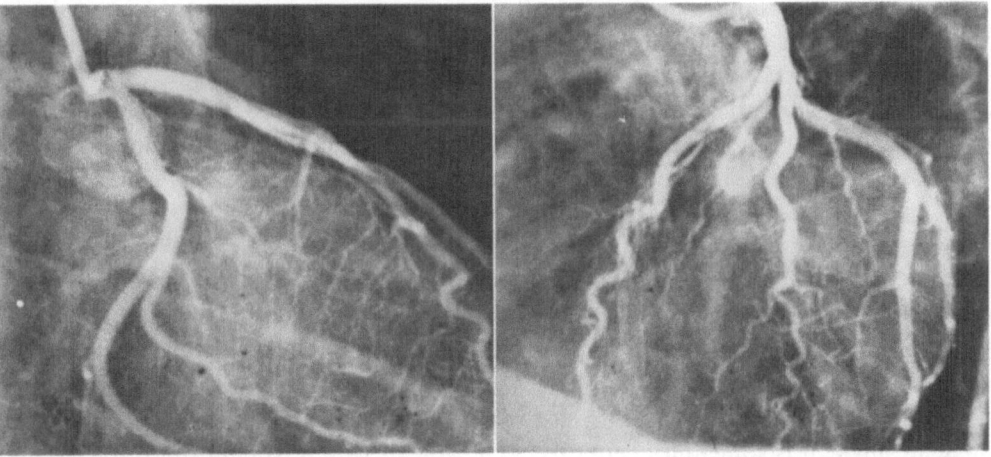

Fig. 6. Normal left coronary artery.
Left: right anterior oblique projection.
Right: left anterior oblique projection.

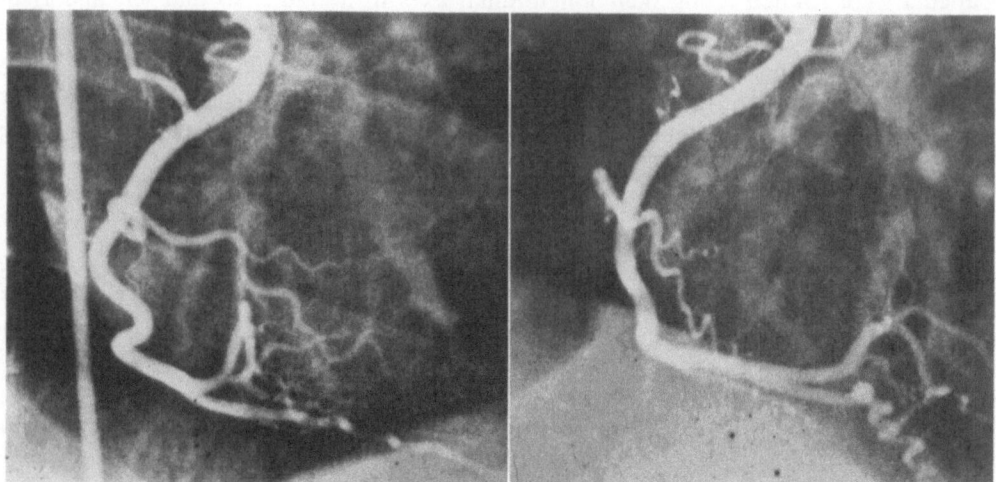

Fig. 7. Normal right coronary artery.
Left: right anterior oblique projection.
Right: left anterior oblique projection.

that an anomaly was present at the posterior part of the heart in which case a radio opaque injection was usually also given to the patient in the left anterior oblique position. If mitral insufficiency was suspected the contrast medium was injected only in diastole with the aid of a R-wave triggered injector (Contraves injector). All 35 mm films were copied onto 16 mm stock and these were evaluated in the usual manner. If required, extra nitroglycerin was administered during the examination and in one instance when a vasovagal reaction was noted a bolus of atropine was given when raising the patient's legs was not effective.

After the angiographic series was finished the patient received 50 mg Protamine chloride intra-arterially and the femoral artery was compressed manually until the bleeding had stopped (minimum fifteen minutes); subsequently a compression bandage was applied to each patient for about twenty-four hours. Originally, in order to re-catheterise the patients use was made of arteriotomy of the brachial artery. Later it was found, however, that the bypasses could also be visualised satisfactorily (figs. 8 and 9) by employing the Seldinger technique (percutaneous approach to the femoral artery). For visualization of the veins, which anastomoses the aorta to the left coronary arteries, the catheter intended for the right coronary artery (Judkins) is a suitable one. In order to find the orifice of the right venous bypass which often branches off the ascending aorta at an acute angle, it is sometimes better to use a catheter with a straight tip. In these latter cases we used a Gensini catheter no. 7 or 8. In all cases where it is deemed necessary, the internal mammary artery can quickly be reached with a special preshaped Cordis-Ducor catheter, type 524-820.

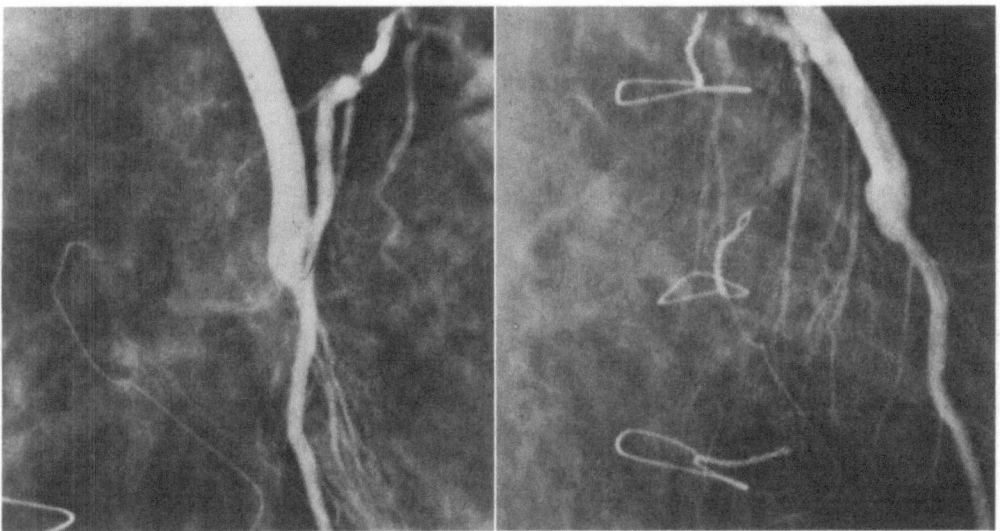

Fig. 8. Normal anastomosis between saphenous vein graft and left anterior descending branch of the left coronary artery.
Left: left anterior oblique projection.
Right: right anterior oblique projection.

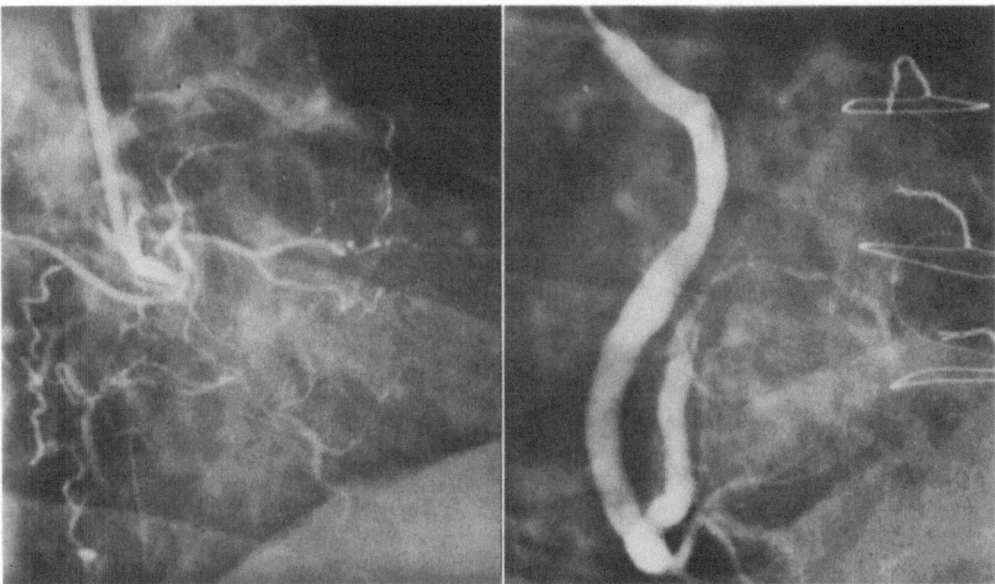

Fig. 9. Left: right coronary artery in right anterior oblique projection. Before operation.
Right: same right coronary artery after bypass procedure.

2.2.6. Diameter of coronary vessels and bypasses

The 70 mm fluorographs were also used for measuring the diameters of the coronary arteries and bypasses. The part to be measured was marked (figs. 11 and 12). In order to obtain the correct diameter, the fluorographs are scanned with a Joyce Loebl microdensitometer. The specimen under view is optically scanned and the variations in density along the scan reproduced on a graph. The X-axis represents the distance along the sample and the Y-axis the density of the sample relative to an internal standard. If the intensities of beams I and II are not equal, the output signal of the photomultiplier tube drives a motor which moves the optical wedge, until both intensities are equal. Mechanically linked to the optical wedge is the recorder pen, the deflection of which corresponds with the density of the specimen (fig. 10). In these cases the scans are made in a direction perpendicular to the veins, arteries and reference points (catheter or wire). The size of the illuminated spot is in the order of 0.05×1.0 mm, the long side being parallel with the vein to be measured. The ratio between recorder and specimen table has in most cases been chosen as 10:1.

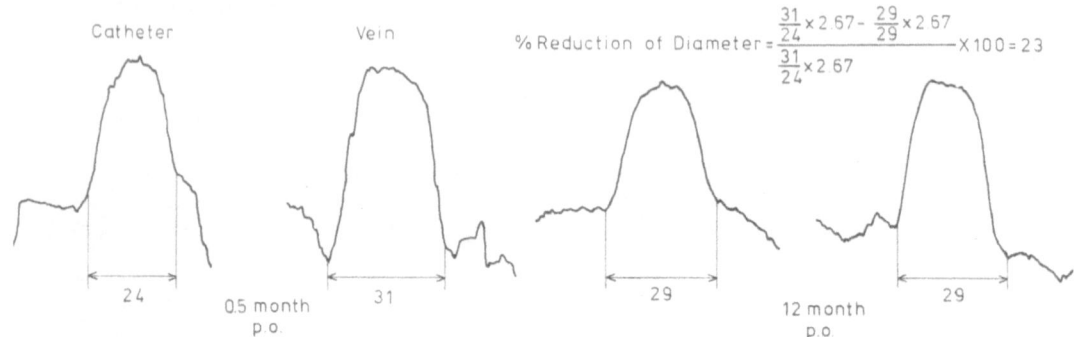

$$\% \text{ Reduction of Diameter} = \frac{\frac{31}{24} \times 2.67 - \frac{29}{29} \times 2.67}{\frac{31}{24} \times 2.67} \times 100 = 23$$

Catheter   Vein

24   0.5 month p.o.   31   29   12 month p.o.   29

Fig. 10. Densitometric scans.

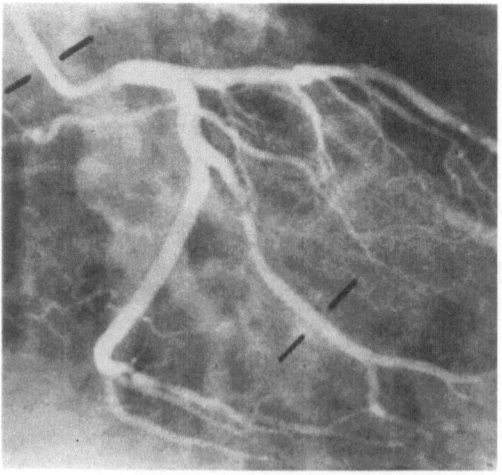

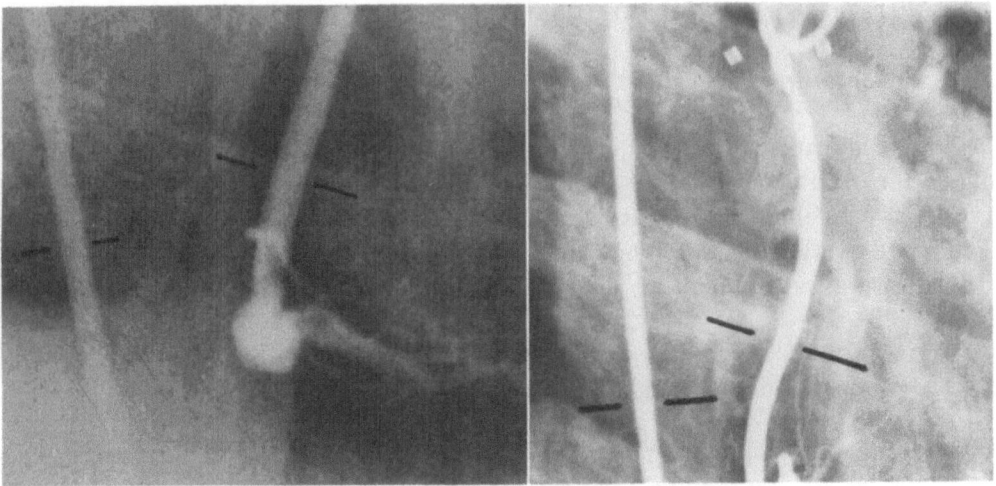

Fig. 12. Saphenous vein graft to right coronary artery in right anterior oblique projection.
Left: direct post-operative.
Right: one year post-operative.

The venous bypasses were visualized and measured two weeks as well as twelve months after operation and care was taken to ensure that the scans were made:
1. on the same place;
2. with the same X-ray beam projection;
3. and that the same reference points were used (fig. 12).

2.3. SURGICAL TECHNIQUE

The operations were performed in the Thoracic Surgical Department of the University Hospital, Leiden. In all patients extra-corporeal circulation was used. Initially the large saphenous vein was taken, but later veins from the lower leg were used. On twelve occasions, instead of a vein, the internal mammary artery was anastomosed with the anterior descending branch of the left coronary artery. Endarterectomy was performed on eight occasions.

In a number of patients, after the proximal and distal anastomosis had been formed the flow through the grafts was measured with the use of an electromagnetic flowmeter; the technique of which has been described by Van der Mark and Frank (1972). The ostia of the veins in the aorta were marked by placing a small metal ring above and below them in order to facilitate post-operative catheterisation (figs. 12, 17, 18, 40 and 41).

← *Fig. 11.* Left coronary artery in right anterior oblique projection. The catheter and coronary artery are scanned between the solid lines.

2.4. TWO PERIODS OF CLINICAL INVESTIGATION

2.4.1. Pre-operative examination

Practically all patients were first examined as out-patients; later hospitalization was required for heart catheterisation and further clinical evaluation. Finally, results of the various examinations were discussed with the staff of the Departments of Cardiology and Thoracic Surgery. After reaching agreement with regard to the indication for surgery, the patient was called up by the Thoracic Surgical Department for admission and operation.

2.4.2. Post-operative examination

Every effort was made to catheterise all patients immediately post-operatively, before leaving the Thoracic Surgical Department. Particular attention was given to visualization of the bypasses, whether they consisted of veins or of the internal mammary artery. Usually, at the immediate post-operative investigation the original (now bypassed) coronary arteries were not visualized, nor was the left ventricular angiogram repeated in the direct post-operative period. This latter was dispensed with, in order to keep the duration of the angiographic examination as short as possible. The patients were discharged from hospital with a maintenance dose of digoxine, in some cases it was given in combination with diuretics. All patients were seen for the first time post-operatively at the out-patients department six to ten weeks after discharge from the hospital and the digoxine therapy was usually discontinued after about three months. Initially all patients were given a maintenance dose of 1 tablet of a long acting nitrate six times per day, but later this routine was abandoned. If nothing special was noted at the first, the second visit to the outpatient department took place six months after discharge, where an exercise-test was added to the usual physical examinations and an 12-lead electrocardiogram. Depending on the patient's general condition, the next examination took place three to six months later and – except for those in whom all grafts had been shown to be closed-up directly post-operatively – we aimed at performing a complete catheterisation in all patients twelve months after operation, i.e. coronary angiography, left ventricular angiography and angiography of the bypasses.

We felt that we owed our patients an explanation for these investigations and pointed out that in the first place it is very important for their own well being to ascertain the condition of the new vessels while, secondly, the information so obtained is valuable for patients who have yet to be operated on. Only three patients refused to be catheterised immediately after the operation as well as one year later, and only three patients refused the second re-examination. The medication of the patients was adapted to their individual needs; all were given anticoagulants, however. When serum lipids proved to be abnormally high a low-fat diet was prescribed, combined in a number of cases with colifibrate.

If patients post-operatively had angina, the same routine treatment was given as was done pre-operatively. Thus, in addition to nitroglycerin a beta-blocker was prescribed and digoxin was given when necessary.

CHAPTER 3

RESULTS OF BYPASS SURGERY

Summary

This chapter deals with results of the operations and the examinations. The overall mortality for 103 operations in 100 patients was 9.7 per cent. An abnormal electrocardiogram was found in 22% of those patients who underwent aorto-coronary bypass surgery only. The direct patency rate of the grafts was 83% and the late patency rate 74%. In veins connecting the aorta with the left circumflex artery patency rate was lower than in veins which bypassed the anterior descending- or the right coronary artery. In the immediate post-operative angiogram it was shown that occlusions in the grafts as well as in the bypassed coronary arteries, were occasionally seen. Evaluation of late post-operative results showed that of the patients in whom not a single graft was patent, none had shown an improvement in symptoms. In 24 of the 47 patients in whom at least one bypass was patent, the parameters of the exercise-electro-cardiogram were found to be improved 6 months post-operatively. In 12 of the 38 patients who were catheterised 12 months post-operatively, the left ventricular wall on angiography proved to have diminished contractile movements; in 4 of the 38 patients an improved contraction pattern was seen and in 22 there were no demonstrable changes seen in the LV angiogram. 3 Patients sustained a definite myocardial infarction in the late follow-up phase. The 8 patients who died during the last follow-up phase all had had an abnormal left ventricular angiogram prior to the operation.

3.1. DIRECT EVALUATION

Direct evaluation is understood to cover the results and complications which occur during the operation or in the immediate post-operative period while the patient is still in the hospital.

3.1.1. Mortality

In group I, comprising forty-seven patients all having angina pectoris, but with a normal left ventricular angiogram, three patients, or 6 per cent, died during the operation or immediately afterwards (table 1). In cases where the contraction pattern of the left ventricle was abnormal, mortality rose to 15 per cent. Of the seventeen patients (group IV) subjected to aneurysmectomy as well as bypass surgery, two (11%) died. The overall operative mortality in one-hundred and three operations was ten, i.e. almost 10 per cent.

The values of the end-diastolic pressure in the left ventricle are given in table 2 which was compiled in order to ascertain whether this pressure was of prognostic value for the mortality. For patients in groups I to III it appeared that there was no difference in end-diastolic pressure between those who died and those who survived. In group IV – patients with a ventricular aneurysm – the enddiastolic pressure in those who survived was even higher than in those who died. An investigation was also made to assess whether the number of grafts to be made had any influence on the direct mortality. It was found that the direct-operative mortality for a triple bypass was lower (5.5%) than for a single (7.1%) and double bypass operations (11.4%), table 3.

Table 2. Relation between direct mortality and mean left ventricular end-diastolic pressure.

LVED = left ventricular end-diastolic.

Group	Nr. Operation	Mean LVED mm Hg
I – III	81	12
Survivors	74	13
Death	7	12
IV Tot.	17	19
Survivors	15	20
Death	2	15

Table 3. Direct mortality related to single, double or triple bypass procedures (81) in 79 patients. Group I, II and III.

	Nr. Operations	%	Bypass procedure						
			single	%	double	%	triple	%
Survivors	74		26		31		17	
Death	7		2		4		1	
Total	81	8.6	28	7.1	35	11.4	18	5.5

Table 4. Electrocardiographic infarction in relation to direct patency-rate in 69 patients (Group I-III).

ECG	Number of patients	Bypass direct post-operative	
		All patent	At least one occluded
Unchanged	54	44	10
Changed	15 22 %	4 8%	11 52 %
Total	69	48	21

3.1.2. Electrocardiographic changes

Electrocardiographic changes are understood in this connection to be the occurrence of a pathological Q-wave or a bundle branch block. Table 4 reviews sixty-nine of the seventy-two patients (groups I to III), who were all catheterised directly postoperatively. Seven patients died during or immediately following on the operation. Of the forty-eight patients in whom all grafts were patent, four (8%) showed these electrocardiographic changes. In twenty-one patients in whom one or all grafts were occluded, these changes occurred eleven times (52%). This is a significant difference (P = 0.01).

To investigate whether the perfusion time and the time during which the aorta was clamped were related to the electrocardiographic changes, these parameters have been processed and are shown in table 5.

Table 5. Duration of extra corporeal circulation and total clamping time of the aorta (minutes) in relation to electrocardiographic changes.
EC   = extra corporal.
ECG = electrocardiogram.
Ao.Cl. = total clamping time of the aorta.

ECG	1 Bypass		2 Bypasses		3 Bypasses.	
	E.C.	Ao.Cl.	E.C.	Ao.Cl.	E.C.	Ao.Cl.
Unchanged	90	23 (21)	135	41 (23)	152	58 (10)
Changed	182	29 (5)	148	38 (5)	225	68 (4)

( )nr.Patients

Table 6. Patency-rate directly post-operative.
RC   = right coronary artery.
LAD = left anterior descending coronary artery.
LC   = left circumflex coronary artery.
10 mammary arteries to LAD, 7 patent, 3 occluded.

Bypassed vessel	Nr. grafts	Nr. occluded	% occluded
R C	68	10	15
LAD	47	5	11
L C	30	10	33
Total	145	25	17

If we consider first the sub-group of 26 patients who were given one bypass, then it is found that the 5 with a substantially changed electrocardiogram underwent a much longer perfusion (182 minutes as against 90 minutes). This is likewise applicable to the 14 patients who were given three bypasses; the 4 patients with a changed electrocardiogram underwent a perfusion lasting 225 minutes, whereas those without electrocardiographic changes were given extracorporeal circulation for 152 minutes.

The 5 patients with, and the 23 without post-operative electrocardiographic changes, who had all been given two bypasses underwent perfusion of approximately the same duration (148 minutes as against 135 minutes). Irrespective of whether one, two or three bypasses were made the time that the aorta was clamped off was not significantly different for the sub-groups with or without electrocardiographic changes.

3.1.3. Patency rate

Table 6 reviews one-hundred and forty-five grafts which were examined directly post-operatively. It can be seen that twenty-five of the one-hundred and forty-five grafts were occluded (17%).

If one studies which grafts run the greatest risk of occlusion, little difference is found to exist between a graft to the right coronary artery (15%) and one to the anterior descending branch of the left coronary artery (11%). The graft to the circumflex of the left coronary artery, however, occluded markedly more often. Of the thirty grafts applied to the left circumflex or to a large side-branch of it – the obtuse ramus – ten (33%) were found to be already occluded at direct post-operative examination.

This difference in occlusion rate between grafts to the right coronary artery and the anterior descending branch on the one hand, and the left circumflex on the other, is significant (P = 0.01).

Since it is more difficult to make an anastomosis with a small coronary artery it may be expected that a vein connected to such an artery will have a higher occlusion rate than a vein which is joined to a coronary artery with a wider lumen.

Table 7 shows that in our patients there is a tendency towards a higher occlusion rate of veins anastomosed with coronary arteries having diameters of less than 2-3 millimetres (10 of the 16). When the diameter calculated from the coronary angiogram is greater than 2 millimetres, there is less risk of the bypass being occluded directly post-operatively (12 of the 61). This applied to the entire group of bypasses, both for grafts to the right coronary artery and for grafts to the anterior descending branch of the left coronary artery. Here, again, an exception is formed by the veins connected to the left circumflex. Then the occlusion rate is high, even with the large diameter of the vessel (5 of the 13).

If the distal run-off is good, there is a better chance of the vein remaining patent. The good run-off is reflected in a higher flow-rate, measured during the operation.

Table 8 shows that of the thirty-four grafts with an average flow in excess of 40 ml/min. on direct post-operative examination only two were found to be occluded (6%). At an average flow-rate of 40 ml/min. or less, eleven of the thirty-one were found to be occluded, an occlusion rate of 35 per cent. This difference is significant.

Table 7. Diameter of 77 bypassed coronary-arteries in relation to direct patency rates of the grafts.
RC   = right coronary artery.
LAD = left anterior descending coronary artery.
LC   = left circumflex coronary artery.

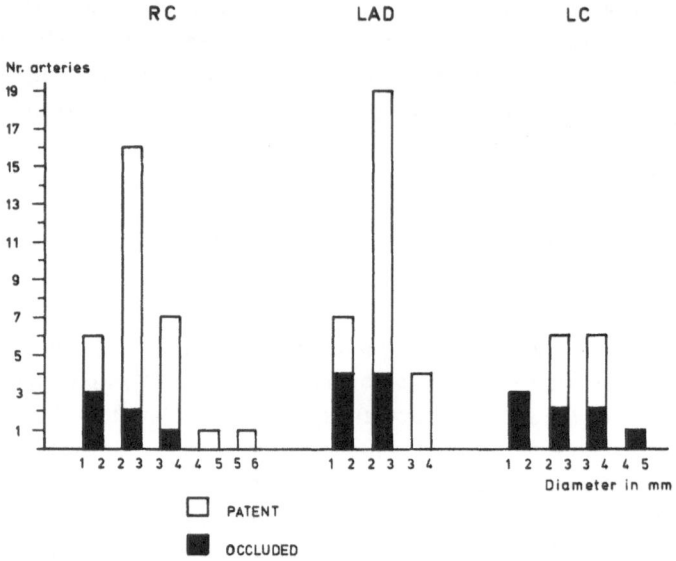

Table 8. Relation between flow-rate and direct post-operative patency-rate.

Mean flow rate	Number of grafts			
ml/min.	Total	Patent	Occluded	%
0 – 40	31	20	11	35
> 40	34	32	2	6
	65	52	13	20

On immediate post-catheterisation stenoses were already found in seven of the one-hundred and forty-five bypasses (figs. 13 and 45). Besides anomalies in the veins, direct post-operative examination disclosed, in a number of patients, anomalies in the bypassed coronary arteries which had not been present pre-operatively. These changes were localised at the level of the distal anastomosis. Thus in one-hundred and twenty bypassed coronary arteries (table 9) a stenosis, if not a total occlusion, was found to have occurred (figs. 15 to 18 and 37 to 39). The phenomenon was noted mainly in grafts which had been anastomosed with the anterior descending branch. Where a venous bypass was used this occurred in eight of the thirty-five (23%); when the internal mammary artery was anastomosed with the anterior descending branch, this was observed in 43 per cent of the cases. With the right coronary artery this was noted in two of the fifty-eight cases (4%).

Table 9. Stenosis in the bypassed coronaries due to the operation.
RC = right coronary artery.
LC = left circumflex coronary artery.
LAD = left anterior descending coronary artery.
ma = mammary artery.

In 7 out of 145 bypasses a stenosis was present at direct post-operative investigation.

Stenosis	Nr. RC	%	Nr. LC	%	Nr. LAD vein	%	Nr. LAD ma	%	All art.	%
Absent	56		18		27		4		105	
Present	2	4	2	10	8	23	3	43	15	13
Total	58		20		35		7		120	

Coronary arteries

3.1.4. Non cardiac complications

One patient showed signs of grave cerebral dysfunction probably ascribable to an embolism during the operation. One patient suffered occlusion of the femoral artery, as result of direct post-operative re-catheterisation. After removal of the thrombus, the circulation in the leg was completely normal and continued to be so for sixteen months after the operation. No other complications following re-catheterisation have occurred.

3.2. LATE EVALUATION

Late evaluation applies to the period immediately following on the patient's discharge from hospital (after the operation). The follow-up time for sixty-eight patients in groups I to III varied from 1 to 38 months, with an average of 19 months (table 10). The time for groups IV and V varied from 3 to 34 months with an average of 18 months. For the total of eighty-one patients the follow-up time was 19 months.

Table 10. Late follow up period (late deaths excluded).

Patients Group	Nr.		Months post-op. Mean	Range
I - III	68		19	1 - 38
IV - V	13		18	3 - 34
Total	81		19	1 - 38

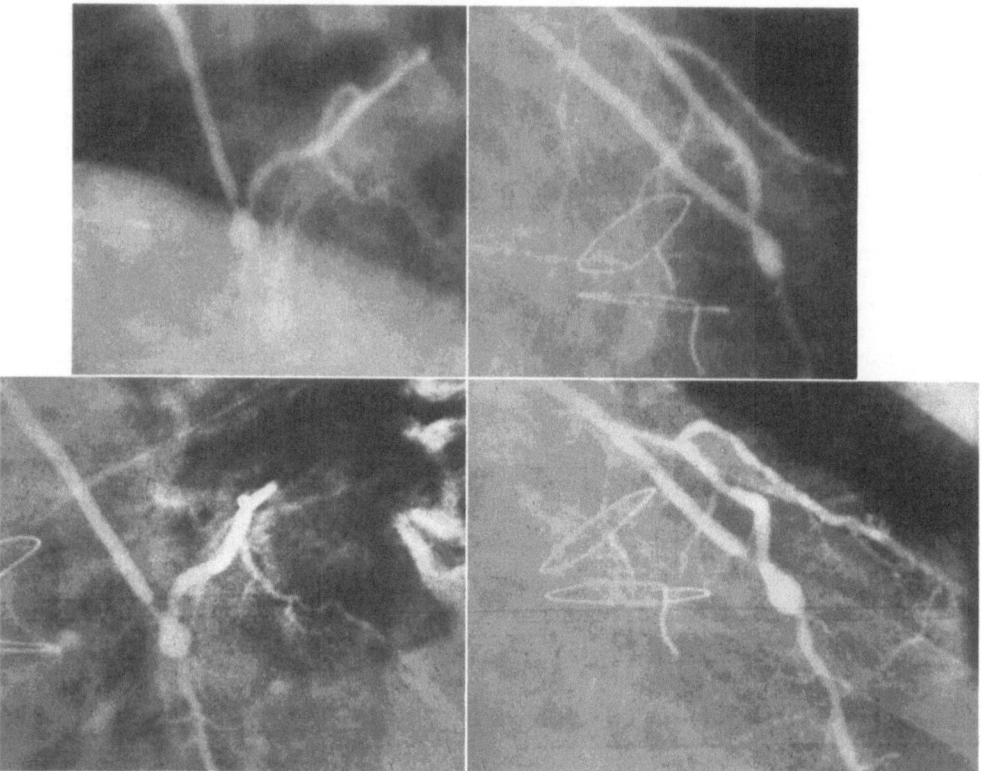

Fig. 13. Saphenous vein graft to left anterior descending with a-stenosis in the end of the graft.
Top left: directly post-operative, left anterior oblique projection.
Top right: directly post-operative, right anterior oblique projection.
Bottom left: one year post-operative, left anterior oblique projection.
Bottom right: one year post-operative, right anterior oblique projection.

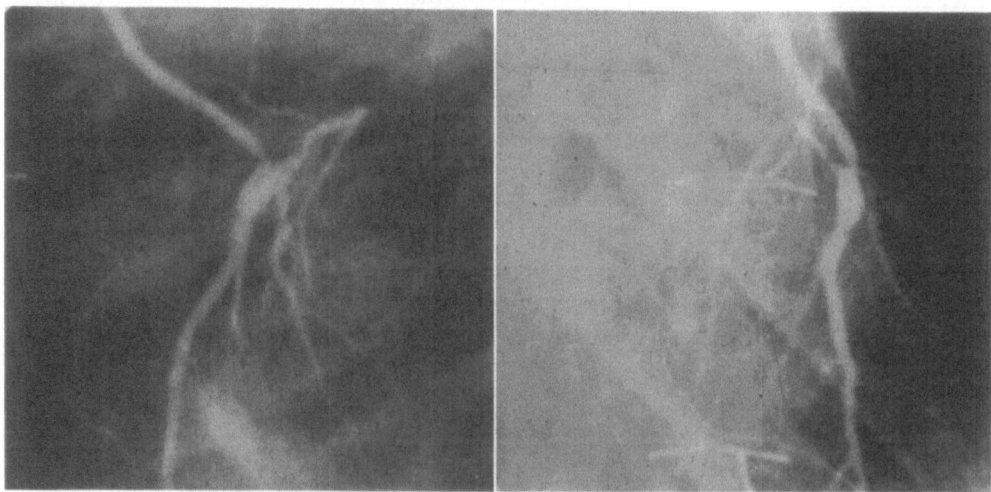

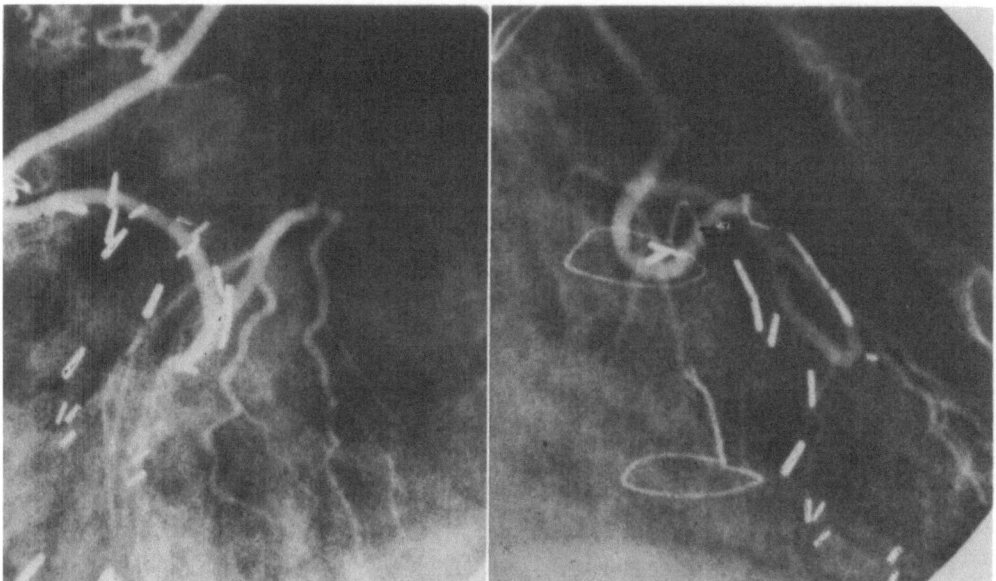

Fig. 15. Left internal mammary artery to the left anterior descending. One year post-operative.
Left: left anterior oblique projection.
Right: right anterior oblique projection.
Note: complete stenosis of the distal part of the recipient artery.

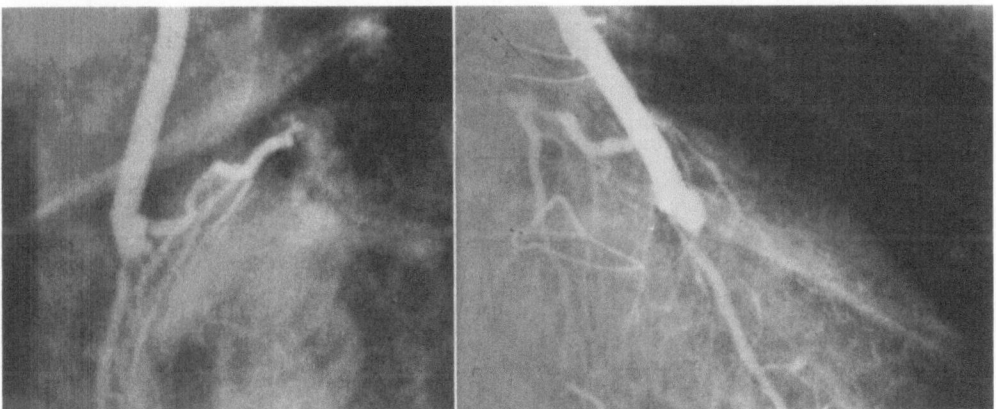

Fig. 16. Saphenous vein graft to the left anterior descending.
Left: left anterior oblique projection.
Right: right anterior oblique projection.
Note: stenosis in the left anterior descending just beyond the distal anastomosis.

← *Fig. 14.* Left internal mammary artery to left anterior descending. One year post-operative.
Left: left anterior oblique projection.
Right: right anterior oblique projection.
Note: stenosis in the mammary artery just before the distal anastomosis, which was also present directly post-operative.

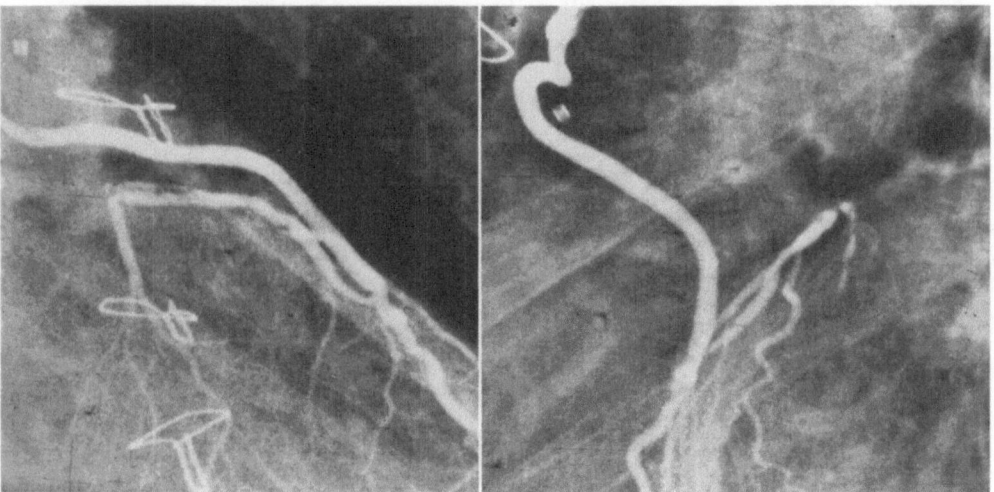

Fig. 17. Saphenous vein graft to left anterior descending. One year post-operative. Normal aspects of the artery and graft.
Left: right anterior oblique projection.
Right: left anterior oblique projection.

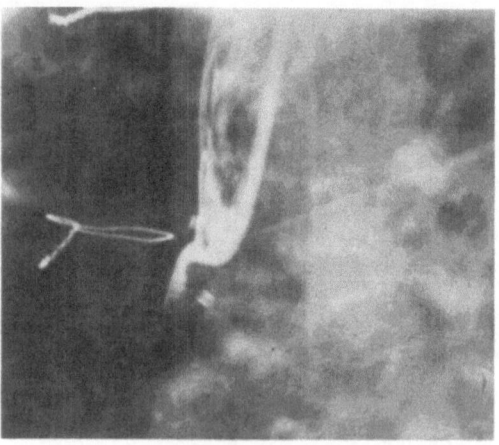

Fig. 18. Saphenous vein graft to right coronary artery in left anterior oblique projection, occluded, one year post-operative.
Note: two metal rings above and below the prox-imal anastomosis.

3.2.1. Symptoms

Not a single patient showed signs of improvement with regard to symptoms in the group of those in whom all grafts were found to be occluded immediately after the operation. However, in six patients out of the group of 35 patients in whom all grafts were found to be patent direct post-operatively, there was no improvement either. The majority of the patients (35) in whom all grafts were patent, stated that they had clearly fewer, or no complaints at all.

3.2.2. Validity

An estimation of the validity provided a somewhat better means of assessing the result of the operation, since then the emphasis lies more on the patient's physical performance.

In table 11 the validity of forty-eight patients prior to the operation is plotted against the validity six months after. All patients had at least one patent bypass. This refers to patients in groups I to III. The numbers of patients in the areas to the left of the diagonal have come into a better group as regards validity. Thus, six of them who were pre-operatively classified as validity group IV, moved up into validity group I six months after operation. Seventeen patients were promoted from validity group III to group I. This implies that of these forty-eight who had undergone surgery, twenty-three were without symptoms six months after the operation. Sixteen patients still complained of symptoms, although less than pre-operatively. Nine patients were classified six months afterwards in the same validity group as they had been in prior to the operation.

Table 11. Validity in 48 patients, a half year post-operative with at least one bypass patent. Group I-II-III.

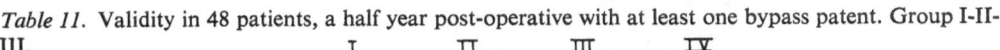
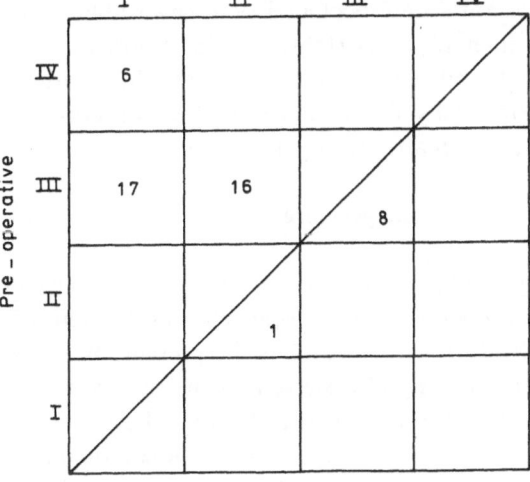

Post-operative.

3.2.3. Exercise electrocardiogram

In my view an important parameter for assessing the result of the operation is the exercise electrocardiogram.

Besides the presence or absence of angina symptoms, the following are important: the maximum load achieved, the degree of S-T depression and, possibly, the product of heart rate and systolic blood pressure (H.R. × B.P.s).

After a successful bypass operation it may be expected that during the exercise test:

1. there should be no angina symptoms, except under very heavy load;
2. the S-T depression should disappear or be less pronounced;
3. the maximum load should be higher than before the operation;
4. the maximum load should be reached at a higher value of the heart rate-systolic blood pressure product (H.R. × B.P.s).

It was not possible to make pre- and post-operative comparisons in all our patients. This was possible, however, in forty-seven patients, and in twenty-one of them all parameters were found to have improved. In contrast to the situation before the operation, twenty-four of the forty-seven no longer had angina during the test. After a successful operation the maximal performance is higher as a rule (table 12). The two patients in whom the maximum performance decreased, stopped the test owing to total exhaustion; this is a change from their reason for stopping the test before the operation when they had to give up because of angina.

Patients in whom all grafts were occluded were never able to surpass their maximum performance by more than 15 watts (table 12). In contrast to the situation before the operation twelve patients showed no electrocardiographic signs of ischaemia during or after maximum load. Practically all patients, even these with occluded bypasses, achieved a higher H.R. × B.P.s product after the operation.

3.2.4. Left ventricular end-diastolic pressure

It was possible in thirty-eight patients in groups I to III to make comparisons of the pre-operative end-diastolic pressure in the left ventricle and the value obtained one year after the operation (table 13). In fourteen patients the pressure was normal both before and after the operation (0-11 mm Hg). In twelve patients the pressure was elevated both before and after the operation (> 11 mm Hg). In four of the five patients whose pressure changed to abnormal, at least one graft was occluded. In one of the seven patients with a normalised end-diastolic pressure, only one graft was occluded.

Table 12. 47 patients group I-III.

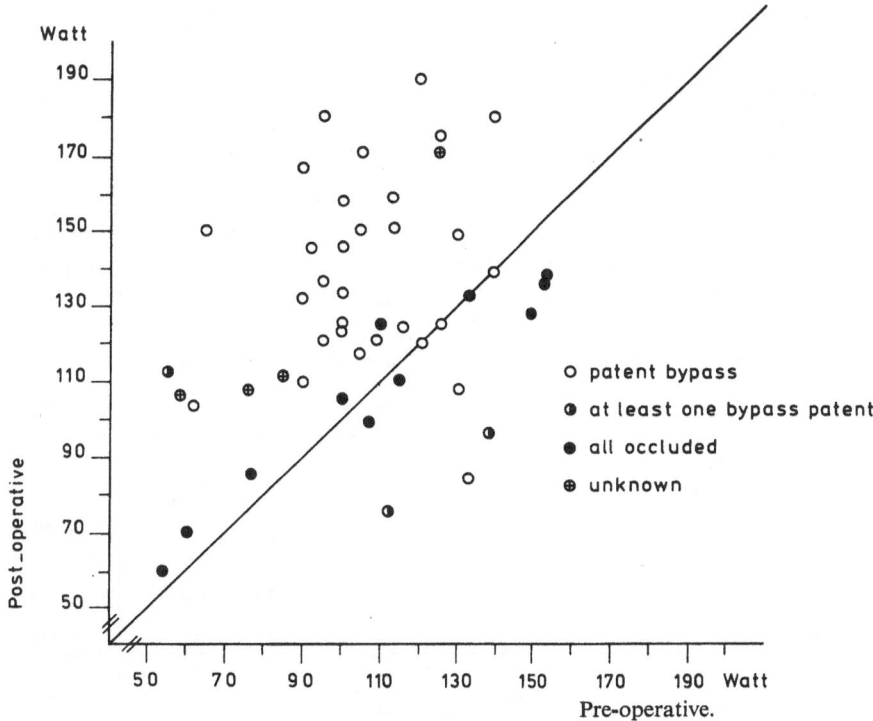

Table 13. Left ventricle end-diastolic pressure in 38 patients before and one year after the operation. Group I-III.

Pre-operative.

		Normal	Abnormal
Post_operative	Normal	14	7
	Abnormal	5	12

3.2.5. Patency rate

Table 14 shows how many of the grafts that were originally patent were found to have sludged after one year. For grafts on to the right coronary artery this occurred in 9/35, i.e. 26 per cent of cases.

As regards the left coronary artery there is a difference between grafts to the anterior descending branch and grafts to the left circumflex. In this latter case an occlusion rate of four of eleven, i.e. 36 per cent, was found, whereas the rate was much lower for grafts to the anterior descending branch, viz. five of twenty-three, i.e. 22 per cent. In the direct post-operative evaluation as well as in the evaluation of the results one year post-operatively a relation was found between flow-rate (measured during operation) and patency. At an average flow of 0-40 ml/min. the occlusion rate was 33 per cent, while at a higher flow this value dropped to 21 per cent (table 15).

An excessively high serum cholesterol level often accompanies coronary sclerosis; one can, therefore, ask whether the serum cholesterol content has any influence on the patency rate. In our series, however, no difference in average serum cholesterol content could be demonstrated in patients in whom the bypasses were patent or in those in whom one or all bypasses were occluded: 290 mg% and 291 mg% respectively.

Table 14. Patency rate 9-32 months post-operative in grafts which were patent directly post-operative.

Mean follow up in months	Bypassed vessel	Nr. grafts	Nr. occluded	% occluded
14	R C	35	9	26
11.5	L A D	23	5	22
14	L C	11	4	36
	Total	69	18	26

Table 15. Relation flow-rate to patency rate one year post-operative in grafts which were patent directly post-operative.

Mean flow-rate ml/min	Number of grafts			
	Total	Patent	Occluded	% occluded
0 - 40	15	10	5	33.3
> 40	24	19	5	21
	39	29	10	26

3.2.6. Changes in the veins

In a number of patients changes were found in the veins or in the internal mammary artery one year after the operations.

These changes can be classified into:

– local stenoses;
– generalised abnormalities.

Table 16 shows that such a local stenosis occurred in six of fifty-one veins (12%). These changes were found in veins running both to the right and to the left coronary arteries. Some examples are shown in figs. 40, 41 and 42. In one patient such a stenosis which was present in the proximal as well as the distal end of the vein, necessitated a repeat operation. We apply the term generalised abnormalities when the lumen of the vein has diminished over the entire length. We observed this mainly in the case of grafts applied to the right coronary artery (fig. 39).

Of all the veins which could be measured directly after, and one year after the operation, it was found that the average diameter had decreased by 26 per cent with a variation of 2 to 60 per cent. The decrease in diameter was less in the twelve grafts running to the left coronary artery. It is striking that practically no changes were observed in the internal mammary artery when used as a bypass. In only one patient a reduction of 7 per cent was found. The decrease in diameter of the veins to the anterior descending branch and that to the left circumflex was 9.4 and 25.6 per cent respectively.

Patients with a serum cholesterol content higher than 300 mg had no greater tendency towards decreased calibre than those in whom the content was lower. The number of grafts measured was, however, small.

Table 16. Localized stenosis in vein grafts one year post-operative.
RC   = right coronary artery.
LAD = left anterior descending.
LC   = left circumflex coronary artery.

	Veins to							
	RC	%	LAD	%	LC	%	All veins	%
Normal nr.	23		16		6		45	
Abnormal nr.	3	12.0	2	11.0	1	14.0	6	12.0
Total nr.	26		18		7		51	

3.2.7. Left ventricular angiogram, electrocardiographic changes and proximal coronary artery

Table 17 shows the relationship between the changes observed in the left ventricular angiogram, electrocardiogram and the proximal coronary artery one year after the operation. In twelve patients the contractions one year later had clearly deteriorated as compared with the situation before the operation; in five of these patients this was not shown in the electrocardiogram. On two occasions a change was found in the electrocardiogram without the ventricular angiogram giving evidence of a situation differing to that prior to the operation. For the time being a well-defined relationship between the three parameters is difficult to discern.

It does not seem very likely that a stenosis in the proximal coronary artery becoming complete might be the cause of the changed contraction pattern in the left ventricle. It is probable, however, that the sludging of the bypass is an important factor in the occurrence of changes in the electrocardiogram (table 4). While the left ventricular contraction may remain unchanged or deteriorate, it is also possible that the contraction pattern will show an improvement. This happened in four patients who all had patent bypasses.

Table 17. 38 patients reinvestigated after one year. Changes in electrocardiogram, left ventricular angiogram and proximal coronary artery.

LEFT VENTRICLE ANGIO
38

		Unchanged		Changed		
		26		12		
		ELECTROCARDIOGRAM				
		Unchanged	Changed	Unchanged	Changed	Total
PROXIMAL COR. ART.	Unchanged	14	1	1	1	17
	Changed	10	1	4	6	21
	Total	24	2	5	7	38

3.2.8. (Re)infarction

Three patients who were all classified pre-operatively in group I, sustained a myocardial infarction in the late follow-up phase, assessed according to the history of pain, electrocardiographic changes and rise in level of serum enzymes. Two patients recovered well after infarction while one made a poor recovery. In all the patients, the bypass was patent immediately after operation, and in one patient this was even the case after one year. In all three the infarction was probably related in some way to occlusion of the bypass. This was confirmed angiocardiographically in two patients (table 18).

Table 18. Myocardial infarction in late follow-up period.
o = patent bypass.
p.o. = post-operative.

	Age	Group	Patency_graft	Months p.o.	Recovery
Patient 1	57	I	0	30	good
,, 2	46	I	000	8	poor
,, 3	43	I	0	32	good

3.2.9. Mortality

Eight patients died after being discharged from the department of thoracic surgery (table 19). It is striking that all except one were in groups III to V and that no substantial changes had been noted in the postoperative electrocardiograms when compared to their pre-operative electrocardiograms. One patient's death was most probably ascribable to a rhythmic disturbance; in addition to two bypasses he was given a Björk-Shiley valve in connection with an insufficiency of the aortic valve. The autopsy on one patient who had been given a bypass and a valve in the mitral ring showed extensive thrombotic changes around the artificial valve. A third patient had cardiomyopathy in addition to stenosis of a coronary vessel. The patient who died twenty-four months after the operation had been pre-operatively classified in validity group IV and had suffered from regular attacks of pulmonary oedema. Three bypasses had been applied in this latter patient; two of them were found to be patent directly post-operatively and also after one year, while an aneurysm of the left ventricle had also been removed.

Table 19. Late deaths – 8 patients.
p.o. = post-operative.

	Age	Group	Patency_graft	Months p.o.
Patient 1	58	II	x o	11
,, 2	55	III	x o	3
,, 3	52	III	o	25
,, 4	43	IV	o	4
,, 5	66	IV	oox	24
,, 6	52	IV	x	11
,, 7	61	IV	o	11
,, 8	57	V	oo	4

o=Patent Bypass(direct p.o.)

x=Occluded Bypass(direct p.o.)

Two patients had extensive anterior wall infarction, possibly on the basis of occlusion of the vein bypassing the anterior descending branch of the left coronary artery, while in both instances the direct post-operative result assessed according to the history and the exercise test was not satisfactory. Two patients with a bypass to the right coronary artery and with resection of an aneurysm of the left ventricle expired suddenly; in one the graft was patent directly post-operatively, while in the other it was occluded. In neither instance was there increased stenosis in the bypassed coronary arteries (fig. 19).

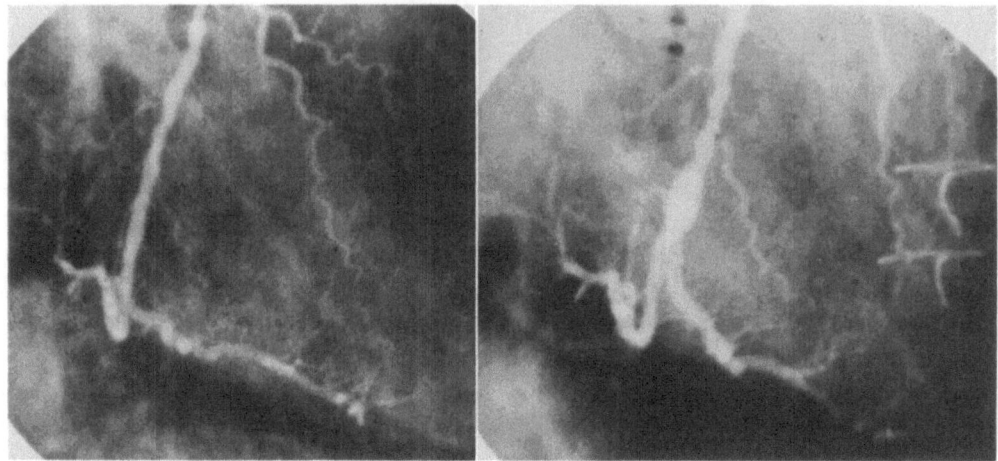

Fig. 19. Right coronary artery after an unsuccesful bypass procedure, right anterior oblique projection.
Left: right coronary artery before the operation.
Right: right coronary artery after the operation.
Note: widening of the artery at the level of the distal anastomosis.

CHAPTER 4

DISCUSSION

Summary

The object of this investigation was to analyse pre-operative, immediate and late post-operative (invasive and non-invasive) cardiac investigations in order to arrive at a selection of patients for aorta-coronary bypass surgical intervention and to provide the surgeon some guidance as to the choice of surgical techniques.

One of our main conclusions is, that when patients dit not improve post-operatively, in some cases it was likely that their symptoms did not arise from coronary sclerosis. Secondly, it was also found that occasionally coronary arteries were narrowed not only at the proximal, but also at the distal part of the vessels, when little good could have been expected from the bypass operation. Thirdly, the coronary angiograms in some instances depicted gracile distal arteries, which technically rendered effective anastomosis impossible. It could have been foreseen that the blood flow through the bypassing veins would be extremely little. In the fourth place – retrospectively – when looking at the left ventricular angiograms and judging the LV function it could be concluded that in a few given patients the myocardium was clearly so severely damaged prior to operation that hardly any improvement from increased coronary flow could have been expected. The described analysis of the observations on bypass operations gave rise to some advice as regards modifications in surgical techniques used in our clinic. Probably as a result of this in the second half of 1973 and the first half of 1974 fewer local obstructions in grafts as well as coronary arteries were seen immediately and late post-operatively. Also patency rate improved in the second half and it can then be expected that also late patency rate will be improved since there is positive correlation between early and late results in patency rate. It should be noted, however, that by-passing veins to the circumflex artery and its main branch – the ramus obtusus – at least in our series, are more inclined to become obstructed than the veins to the right coronary artery or the left anterior descending coronary artery. In 82% patients angina pectoris symptoms diminished or disappeared post-operatively. This figure is in agreement with results reported from other centres and underscores that aorta-coronary bypass surgery for patients with angina pectoris predictably relieves disability from angina. In 6 instances patients were operated upon for the type of progressive angina, all of whom improved as regards symptoms, from the operation. In the past, relief of angina has been attributed to many other surgical methods which later could be proven not to really increase blood flow to the myocardium. In the case of the aorto-coronary bypass technique the relief of disability from angina very often is accompanied by normalization or improvement in objective tests, such as electrocardiographic stress tests as was also the case in our series. It can therefore be stated that the aorta-coronary bypass treatment for coronary heart disease is probably an effective method, and in that respect it differs from all previous attempts to surgically treat angina pectoris. However, in order to be able to recommend this type of operation to a greater number of patients it also is required to investigate what effects the aorto-coronary bypass surgical intervention has on the patient's lifetime expectancy and on the risk, the operated patients run of sustaining myocardial infarction. In other words, the natural history of the aorto-coronary bypass should be studied in carefully planned follow-up studies, preferably of the type in which randomisation of the patients is applied.

4.1. OBJECT OF BYPASS OPERATION

The object of the saphenous vein bypass operation is:

– to alleviate the patient's distress if not to eliminate it;
– to reduce the risk of (re)myocardial infarction;
– to increase the patient's life expectancy.

When analysing the results achieved with the saphenous vein bypass operation the first objective is the easiest to evaluate. One can ask the patient whether he or she feels that his or her angina symptoms have subsided after the operation, and in many cases the answer will be in the affirmative. It is not enough, however, to measure the value of the operation against the yardstick of a changed symptomatology. For instance, the majority of patients who undergo sham operations consider their condition to have improved.

With our patients, too, it was striking that some stated they had fewer symptoms after the operation, although objective (excercise test and post-operative angiogram) examination indicated no improvement. Of all revascularization operations the bypass procedure is the first for which an improvement can be objectively demonstrated. Little is known of what effect the operation may have on:

– the patient's life expectancy;
– the risk of a myocardial infarction.

Large series of patients in whom all relevant data are known are rare. In 1972 Sheldon et al. published data on one-thousand patients who had undergone surgery; he compared the annual mortality in this series with that for another series of patients who had had angiocardiographic abnormalities but who had not been operated on. For those in the first series the annual mortality was 4.1 per cent, including death during the operation. In the patients not treated surgically the annual mortality was 6.8 per cent (5 year follow-up). These figures do not, however, warrant the conclusion that an operation increases the life expectancy since, after all, the groups of patients who were compared with each other – surgery versus medical treatment – were not chosen at random. Under ideal circumstances, every new therapy of uncertain value should be subjected to randomization. Medicine is, however, not a science to which only strict scientific criteria can be applied.

If a patient with severe symptoms asks for help it is understandable that one will consider an operation, the risk being willingly accepted by the patient, if experience has shown that it has a good chance of alleviating the symptoms. It is this very insistance on the part of the patients to have an operation, that creates a situation in which randomization is almost impossible.

In comparison with those treated in the large American Clinics, our patients are small in number, but in view of the many factors which can determine the results of the operation every centre should subject the results and complications to a careful investigation, so that in this way each can establish:

– reliable indications;
– a guide to the choice of surgical technique.

4.2. ESTABLISHMENT OF INDICATION

The pillars on which the diagnosis of coronary sclerosis rests are:

– history;
– excercise electrocardiogram;
– coronary angiogram;
– left ventricular angiogram.

During the initial period we were not fully aware of the discrepancy that can exist between these pillars. If the patient presented has symptoms which are difficult to interpret, a clinical analysis with extensive heart catheterisation can easily be carried out. If the coronary angiogram indicates certain abnormalities it is tempting to ascribe the symptoms to them. It should not be forgotten, however, that the coronary angiogram is a 'snap-shot' as it were, made at a moment when the patient is usually without symptoms. A slight or even severe stenosis of a coronary artery need not be the cause of ischaemia of the myocardium, and certainly not if the patient is at rest.

Johnson et al. (1969) hold the view that the stenosis should occupy at least 75 per cent of the lumen if surgery is to be justified. This is based on the fact that he could find no pressure gradient over the stenosis if it was less than 75 per cent. These pressure differences over the constriction are measured, however, at rest and during the operation. It is important to know what influence a stenosis in the coronary arteries has on the blood supply to the myocardium under a work load, and which stenosis is likely to increase and which not. In our first series of patients there were some in whom in retrospect it was found that the above-mentioned diagnostic pillars had been incorrectly assessed. In three patients the symptoms after a technically successful operation did not diminish. One patient was troubled by arrhythmia; two others, in addition to coronary sclerosis, probably also had non-obstructive cardiomyopathy. In all three patients the exercise electrocardiogram could not be called positive since S-T depressions were absent and these patients had no typical angina symptoms under maximal work load. They were all given a venous bypass to the right coronary artery which was directly post-operatively patent, but after a year not a single graft was functioning. When the coronary angiogram of one patient was critically scrutinised it was found that he had stenoses not only in the proximal part of the arteries but in the distal parts as well. Two bypasses probably did not help to alleviate the symptoms and both grafts were occluded six months after the operation.

It is doubtful to say the least that this patient should have been operated upon. The age and the end-diastolic pressure in the left ventricle were of little prognostic value for the direct-operative mortality. Of groups I, II and III which comprised forty-seven, twenty and twelve patients respectively, three (6,25%), two (10%) and two (15,3%) died immediately after operation; two were operated upon twice (table 1). These numbers are too small to demonstrate significant differences, but there is a trend indicative of the operative mortality increasing accordingly as the left ventricular angiogram is more abnormal. The higher risk associated with an abnormal left ventricular angiogram can be explained by the fact that the myocardium of these hearts is more damaged and has more extensive or more serious abnormalities than the myocardium of hearts with a normal contraction pattern. If, then, the equilibrium between blood supply and blood demand is disturbed, e.g. as result of surgery, patients in group II and III would enter into a critical condition quicker than those in group 1. Not only is the direct mortality higher, the late mortality also appears to be higher was well (table 19).

Among our patients there is a good correlation between classification in groups I, II and III on the one hand and the number of clinically experienced infarctions on the other. Five of the seven patients who died direct post-operatively did so in the operating room. Their hearts were unable to provide a good blood pressure after the heart lung machine was disconnected. During the operation all five patients showed electrocardiographic signs of ischaemia or myocardial infarction. In four of these seven patients the coronary arteries on to which the vein or the internal mammary artery, as the case may be, had to be connected were of small calibre; approximately 1 to $1\frac{1}{2}$ millimetres cross-sectionally. One patient died of ventricular fibrillation on the fifth day after operation; at post-mortem a thrombus was found in the vein connected to the left anterior descending coronary artery. Another patient died four weeks after operation of forward failure. In judging whether a vessel can be bypassed, it is important to know the distal run-off as well as the diameter. The coronary vessel that supplies blood to a small region of heart muscle tissue only, does not seem worth bypassing, particularly since an occluded bypass increases the risk of a myocardial infarction (table 4).

It is difficult to measure the distal run-off pre-operatively, but it is reflected in the flow measured during the operation. With an average flow rate of less than 40 ml per minute there is greater risk of the vein not only becoming occluded directly after the operation, but also of it occluding in the course of the first post-operative year (table 15).

A properly functioning bypass can occasionally result in the proximal stenosis becoming complete. If the bypass then sludges (which is the case in 18% according to Sheldon et al., 1972), the heart may be worse off than before the operation. In our series it was not possible to correlate the flow rate with the pre-operatively measured diameter of the coronary artery because the flow had not been measured in every patient.

The operative hazard does not seem to have been increased by the number of bypasses as such (table 3). It must be emphasised, however, that the group of patients who had been given one bypass only was not homogeneous, since it included those with two or three diseased vessels, of which only one could be considered as technically suitable for a bypass. Naturally these patients have poorer coronary systems than those who are given one bypass because of the fact that only one vessel is diseased, the other coronary vessels being normal and patent.

Patients with an unstable angina call for a separate discussion; these are the patients whose symptoms become rapidly worse and who sometimes have severe angina even at rest. When medical treatment fails to relieve the symptoms, we have adopted a radical attitude towards these patients, that is: to operate as soon as the coronary angiogram is made. Although one can never be completely certain, we think that these patients did not sustain a myocardial infarction; this is based on the fact that:

– electrocardiographic changes were only of a temporary nature;
– the serum enzymes did not become elevated.

Neither surgery nor coronary angiography gave rise to complications. Three patients had a sub-total (fig. 32) stenosis in the anterior descending branch, three patients had a three vessels disease. Five of the six patients were without symptoms post-operatively; after a follow-up period of at least thirteen months and their exercise tests were negative.

The following descriptions are illustrative of this type of clinical picture. Figures 20 and 21 show left ventricular angiograms immediately prior to operation and twelve months afterwards respectively. Before the operation the anterior wall of the left ventricle was hypokinetic as result of a serous stenosis in the anterior descending branch. After a venous bypass had been applied to this vessel, the left chamber contracted completely normally both immediately after the operation and thirteen months later. The vein remained patent.

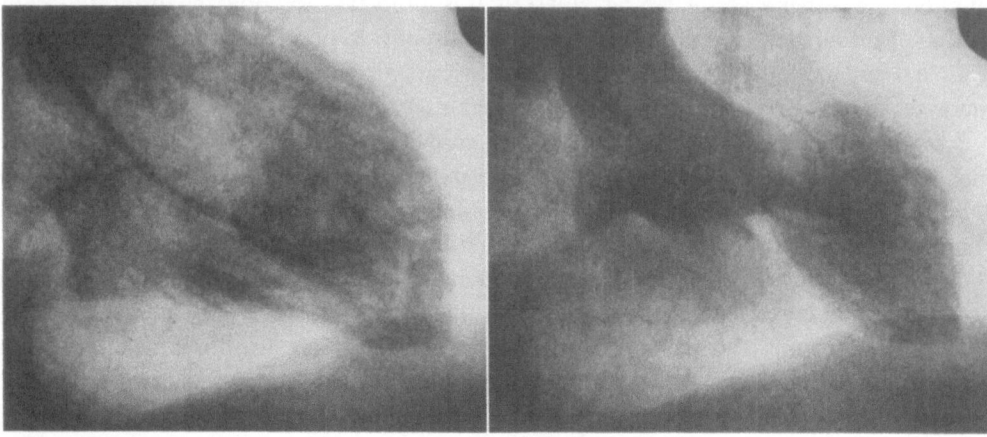

Fig. 20. Left ventricle angio in right anterior oblique projection before operation.
Left: diastolic phase.
Right: systolic phase.
Note: area of hypokinesia around the apex. Same patient as figure 21.

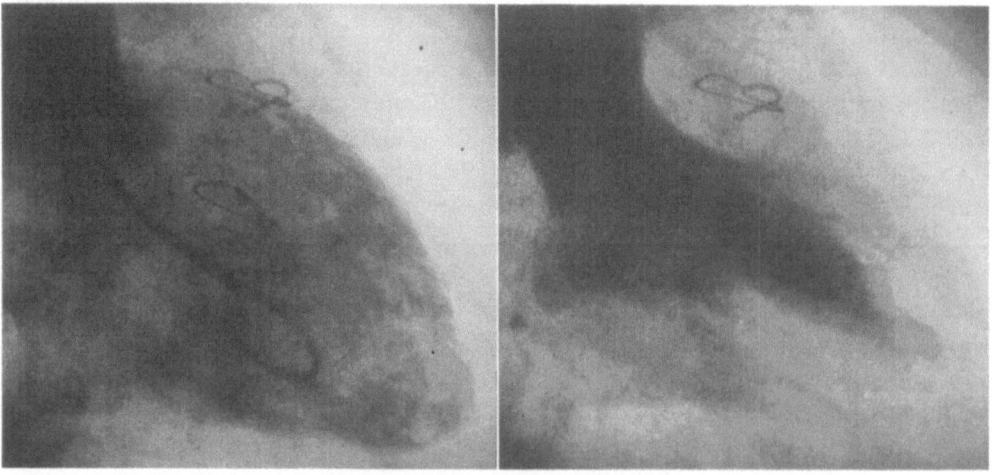

Fig. 21. Left ventricle angio in right anterior oblique projection. 12 months post-operative.
Left: diastolic phase.
Right: systolic phase.
Note: normal wall movements. Same patient as figure 20.

More or less the opposite is presented in figure 22 en 23 which show the left ventricular angiogram of a patient with a sub-total stenosis in the anterior descending branch and who had serious attacks of angina pectoris while at rest; incidentally, this patient reacted well to nitroglycerin. The venous bypass to the anterior descending branch was found to be functioning well direct post-operatively. When followed up after a year the patient was free of symptoms, the exercise electrocardiogram was negative, but the vein was occluded and the left ventricular angiogram showed hypokinesis of the apex.

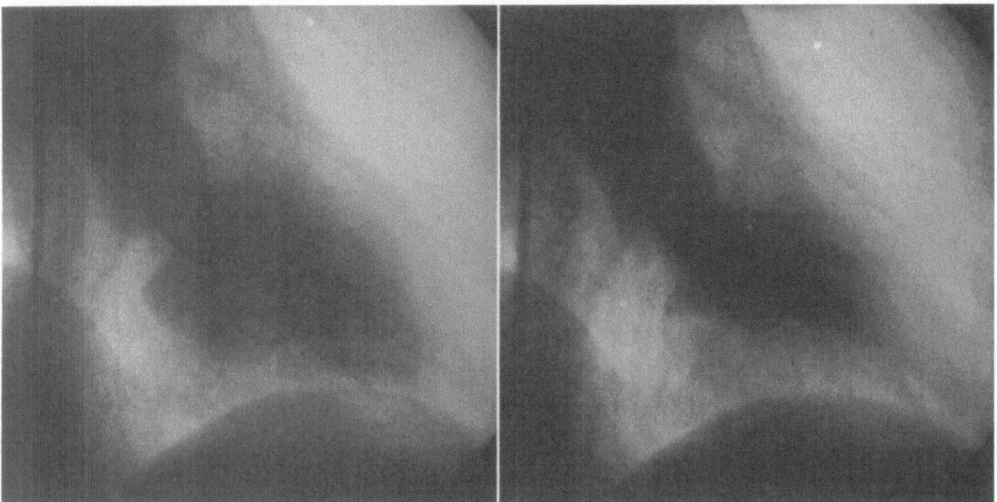

Fig. 22. Left ventricle angio in right anterior oblique projection before operation.
Left: diastolic phase. *Right:* systolic phase.
Note: normal wall movements. Same patient as figure 23.

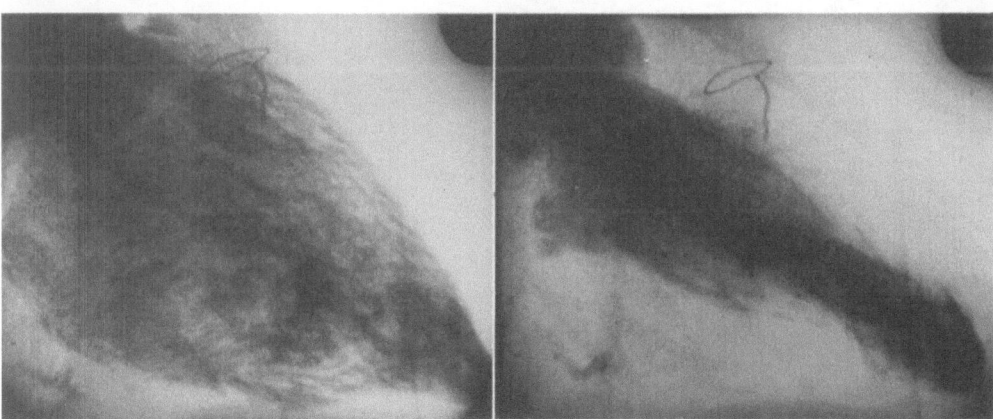

Fig. 23. Left ventricle angio in right anterior oblique projection. 12 months after the operation.
Left: diastolic phase. *Right:* systolic phase.
Note: area of hypokinesia around the apex. Same patient as figure 22.

Figures 24 and 25 show yet another example of a patient who had violent angina attacks at rest, accompanied by S-T elevation and serious arrhythmia. The coronary angiogram showed a serious localised stenosis in the anterior descending branch. The stenosis was bypassed with an internal mammary artery. Twenty-four months later the

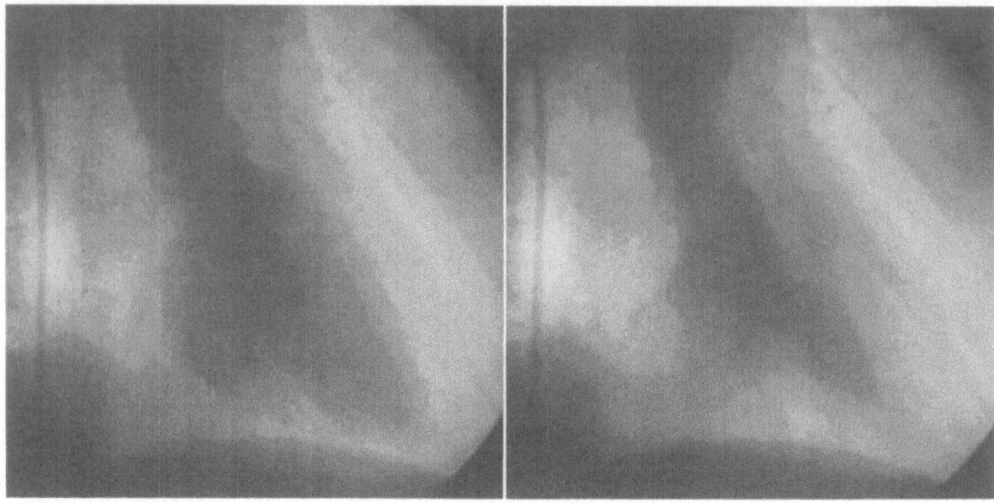

Fig. 24. Left ventricle angio in right anterior oblique projection before operation.
Left: diastolic phase.
Right: systolic phase.
Note: normal wall movements. Same patient as figure 25.

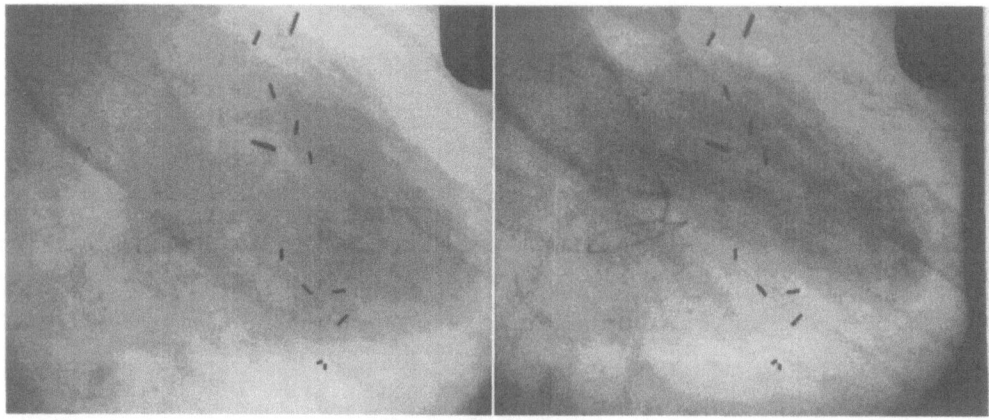

Fig. 25. Left ventricle angio in right anterior oblique projection. 12 months after the operation.
Left: diastolic phase.
Right: systolic phase.
Note: area of hypokinesia of the anterior wall. Same patient as figure 24.

patient is without serious angina symptoms and the exercise electrocardiogram is negative. The anastomosis was functioning well twelve months after the operation, as was also the case direct post-operatively. It is remarkable, however, that the left ventricular angiogram shows a distinct decrease in the motility of the anterior wall, as compared with the situation before the operation. This possibly could be related to the low blood flow through the internal mammary artery.

These examples clearly illustrate that a good pre-operative analysis must be followed up by an extensive post-operative analysis, in order to provide a proper insight into the disease and into the results of the operation.

In our opinion one may not refuse an operation to patients in validity class 4 who are operable; these patients do not, therefore, come into consideration for randomization. We carefully followed up patients with a localised stenosis in one of the coronary arteries who had only moderate symptoms, and in the event of a subjective as well as objective progression of symptoms, we proposed them for operation. Possibly one should consider operation for patients who have a specific type of stenosis, even in the presence of only moderate symptoms. Uncertain factors such as the following, should be studied before a definite attitude towards this problem can be taken:

- which type of venous bypass tends to occlude;
- which stenosis will worsen;
- at what degree of stenosis should a bypass be given;
- in which patients will sufficient collaterals develop (fig. 44).

As regards the exercise electrocardiogram we found that of the forty-seven patients in whom we were able to compare the pre-operative with the post-operative exercise electrocardiogram all parameters had improved in twenty-one. It is very likely that the O_2 supply to the myocardium in these 21 cases had improved. In our series the serum cholesterol content does not appear to have any effect on the patency rate of the by-passing veins one year after operation. From our observations I would tentatively like to conclude that in order to recommend a patient for bypass surgery, there should be:

- typical angina symptoms accompanied with a positive exercise electrocardiographic test;
- distal arteries of approximately 2 mm, and a good distal run-off;
- a normal or only slightly abnormal left ventricular angiogram.

4.3. SURGICAL TECHNIQUE

It is apparent from the literature that in every centre more complications are encountered when a start is made with a new operation than later when experience has been gained. In the series of operations described here hardly any patient was refused operation, particularly not in the early phase. It therefore follows that occasionally operation was carried out on patients with very poor left ventricular function and/or distal stenosis. In ten of the thirty patients who were given a bypassing vein to the left circumflex or to a large side-branch of it, the ramus obtusus, the vein appeared to be occluded already immediately after the operation. The occlusion rate for the grafts to the right coronary artery and the anterior descending branch of the left coronary artery was ten of sixty-eight (15%) and five of forty-seven (11%) respectively. As some examples may clearly show, care should be exercised when interpreting these figures:

1. If a patient has been given three bypasses of which two are found to be occluded after one year while one is functioning properly, e.g. a graft to the anterior descending branch of the left coronary artery, it may well be that this patient has nevertheless benefitted greatly from the operation.
2. Figures 26 and 27 show a venous bypass to the obtuse ramus fifteen months after the operation. This patient no longer suffers from angina pectoris, he does his full job and has no angina symptoms at a maximum work load of 150 watts on the bicycle ergometer. Also, in contrast to the situation before the operation, the exercise electrocardiogram shows no sign of ischaemia. This clearly demonstrates that a bypass to the left circumflex, too, can be very useful.
3. Figure 28 shows a bypassing vein to the left circumflex artery; the very first performed by our surgical team. Instead of being applied distally as should have been done, this anastomosis was applied proximally to the stenosis. The coronary angiogram shown, was made twenty-seven months after the operation. The vein is patent and fills the coronary artery; however, when an injection is made into the original coronary artery, not only did the coronary artery fill but there was also retrograde filling of the vein. It seems very likely that this bypassing vein performs no function whatsoever with respect to the blood supply to the myocardium, but it is interesting to see that this vessel is still fully patent twenty-seven months after operation. (The patient feels definitely improved.)

Fig. 26. Left coronary artery with a stenosis in the left circumflex branch.
Before the operation.
Left: right anterior oblique projection.
Right: left anterior oblique projection.

Fig. 27. Same patient as shown in figure 26. 15 months post-operative.
Left: left coronary artery in right anterior oblique projection.
Right: saphenous vein graft to obtuse branch.

Fig. 28. Saphenous vein graft to left circumflex coronary artery with distal anastomosis before the stenosis in the coronary artery. 26 months post-operative.
Left: left coronary artery injection, with retrograde filling of saphenous vein graft.
Right: saphenous vein graft injection with complete filling of the left coronary artery.

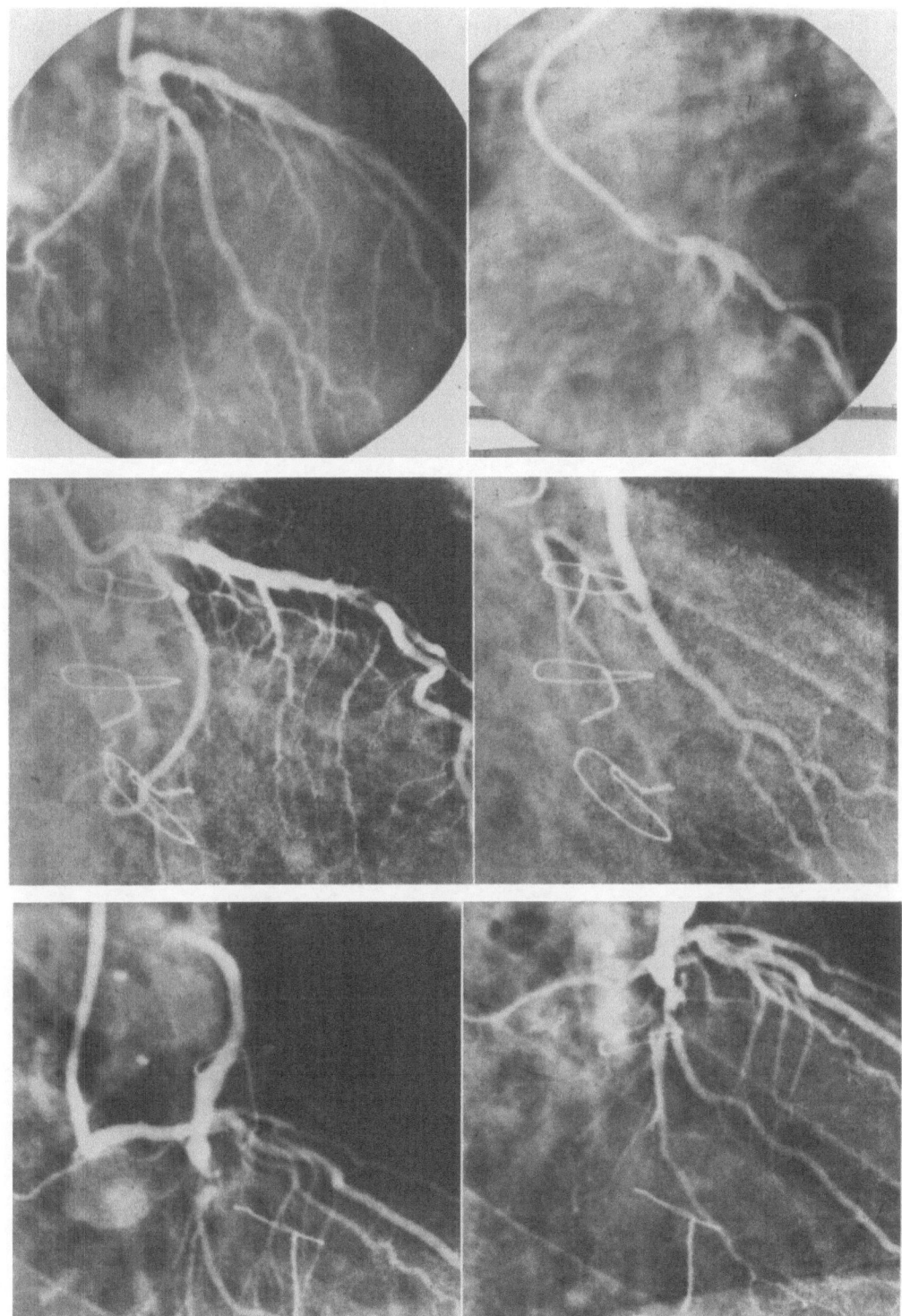

4. Figures 29, 30 and 31 show a bypassing vein to the right coronary artery; this graft was made because of an ostium stenosis which could not be satisfactorily eliminated. Thirteen months after the operation both vein and right coronary artery are adequately patent. When contrast medium was injected into the vein the entire right coronary artery filled, but the reverse is also the case. What the true flow pattern in this vein is, remains uncertain. The patient is entirely without symptoms and has a negative exercise electrocardiographic test, whereas both were positive prior to operation.

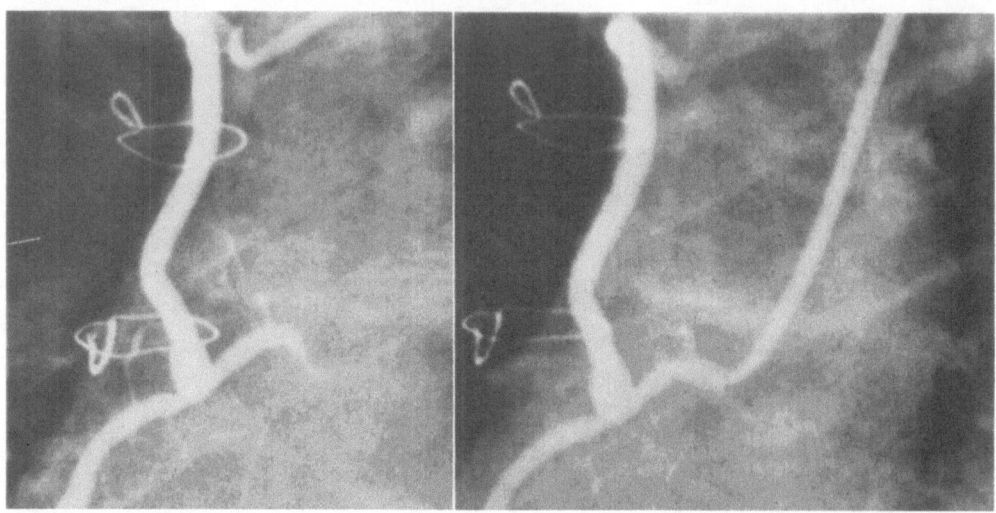

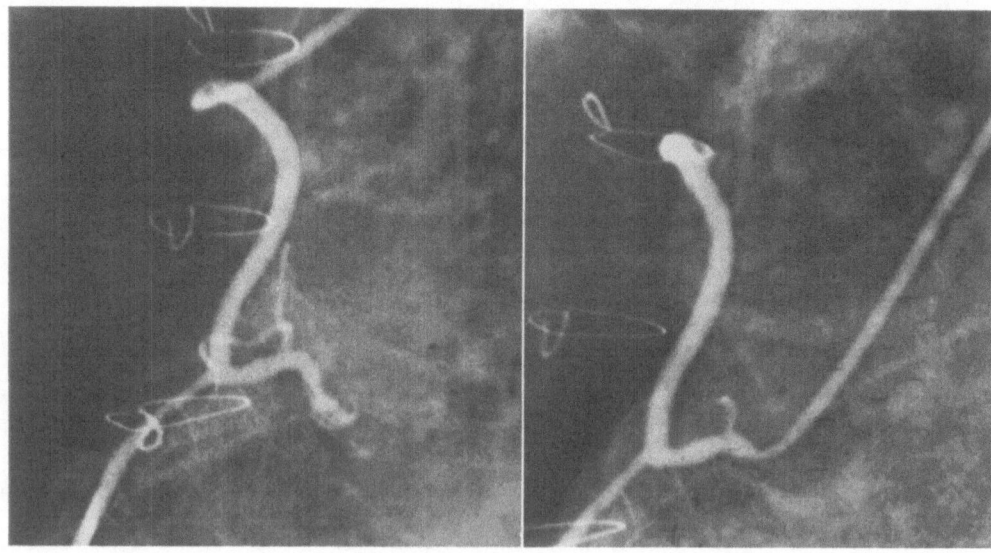

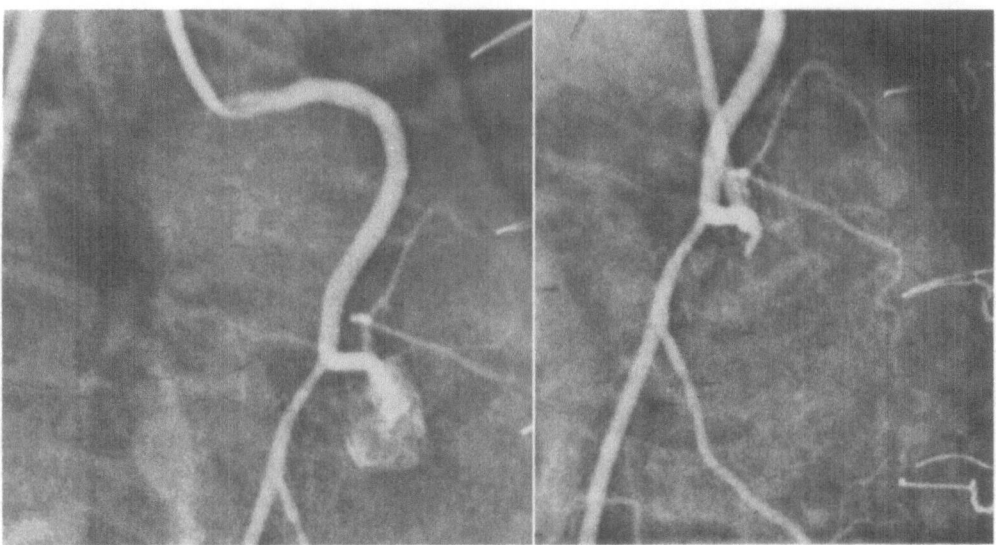

Fig. 31. Saphenous vein graft to right coronary artery. 14 months post-operative. Right anterior oblique projection.
Left: injection in the graft.
Right: injection in the right coronary artery.
Note: same patient as shown in figure 29 and 30. Retrograde filling of the graft.

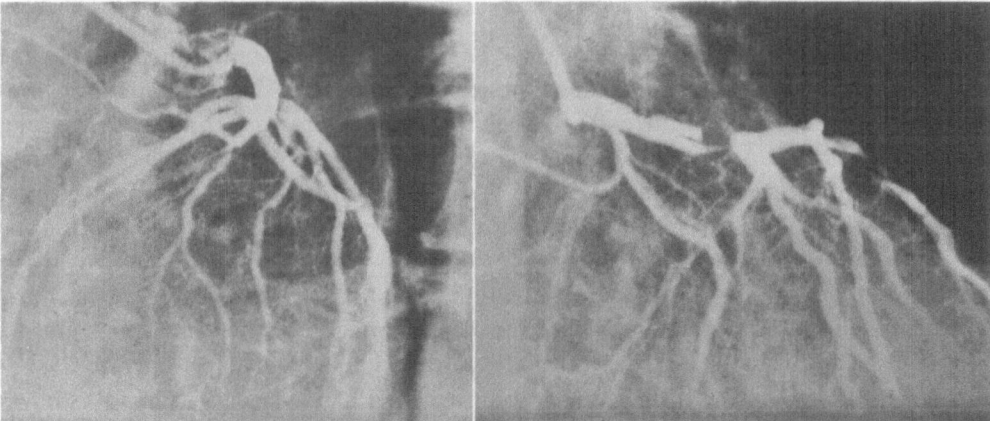

Fig. 32. Left coronary artery with subtotal obstruction of the left anterior descending.
Left: left anterior oblique projection.
Right: right anterior oblique projection.

←   *Fig. 29.* Saphenous vein graft to right coronary artery because of a stenosis of the orifice of the right coronary artery. *Left:* injection in the graft. *Right:* injection in the right coronary artery.
Note: retrograde filling of the graft.

←   *Fig. 30.* Saphenous vein graft to right coronary artery. 14 months post-operative. Left anterior oblique projection. *Left:* injection in the graft. *Right:* injection in the right coronary artery.
Note: same patient as shown in figure 29 and 31.

5. Figure 33 shows a bypassing vein grafted onto a small obtuse ramus, in which the average flow measured during the operation was 30 ml/min. The distal anastomosis is narrow, seventeen months after the operation the vein is still patent and the anastomosis even seems to have become somewhat wider.

A possible explanation for the rather poor results obtained with venous bypasses to the left circumflex artery and to the obtuse ramus is the fact that these coronary arteries are not easily accessible to the surgeon; in other words it is technically more difficult to make a good anastomosis. This is borne out by the fact that the results of operations on this vessel are poor in other centres, too, not only in ours.

Fifteen of our patients in groups I, II and III (69) had significant post-operative electrocardiographic changes. The perfusion time in these patients (table 5) when one and/or three bypasses were being made was much longer than with patients in whom the electrocardiogram was unchanged. The patients who were given two bypasses and who also had electrocardiographic changes had, however, perfusion times which were not longer than those in the patients with two bypasses and unchanged electrocardiograms. The reason for this difference is not clear.

Table 4 shows that an occluded venous bypass increases the probability of the patient having an altered electrocardiogram. An explanation for the high percentage of electrocardiographic changes might be that during the early period we often tried to apply an anastomosis to a too small coronary artery.

When the changes in the left ventricular angiogram, the electrocardiogram and the proximal coronary artery are compared with each other (table 17), the mutual relationships are so complex that no definitive conclusions can be drawn from this small group of patients. On the other hand, when the electrocardiogram clearly indicates that a myocardial infarction has occurred, in seven cases out of nine it is accompanied by a decrease of the wall movements as demonstrated by the left ventricular angiogram. The decrease of wall movement is also seen occasionally without it being reflected in the electrocardiogram by typical Q-wave formation (five of twelve cases). Figure 34 shows an example of such a change in the left ventricular angiogram; the three veins grafted into this patient were satisfactorily patent not only immediately post-operatively but also one year later. In this patient the electrocardiogram showed a right bundle branch block after the operation.

Fig. 33. Saphenous vein graft to the branch over the obtuse margin. Right anterior oblique projection. *Left:* directly post-operative. *Right:* one year post-operative.
Note: narrow distal anastomosis.

Fig. 34. Left ventricle angio in right anterior oblique projection.
Top left: before operation, diastolic phase. *Top right:* before operation, systolic phase.
Bottom left: after operation, diastolic phase. *Bottom right:* after operation, systolic phase.
Note: decreased wall movements 12 months post operative.

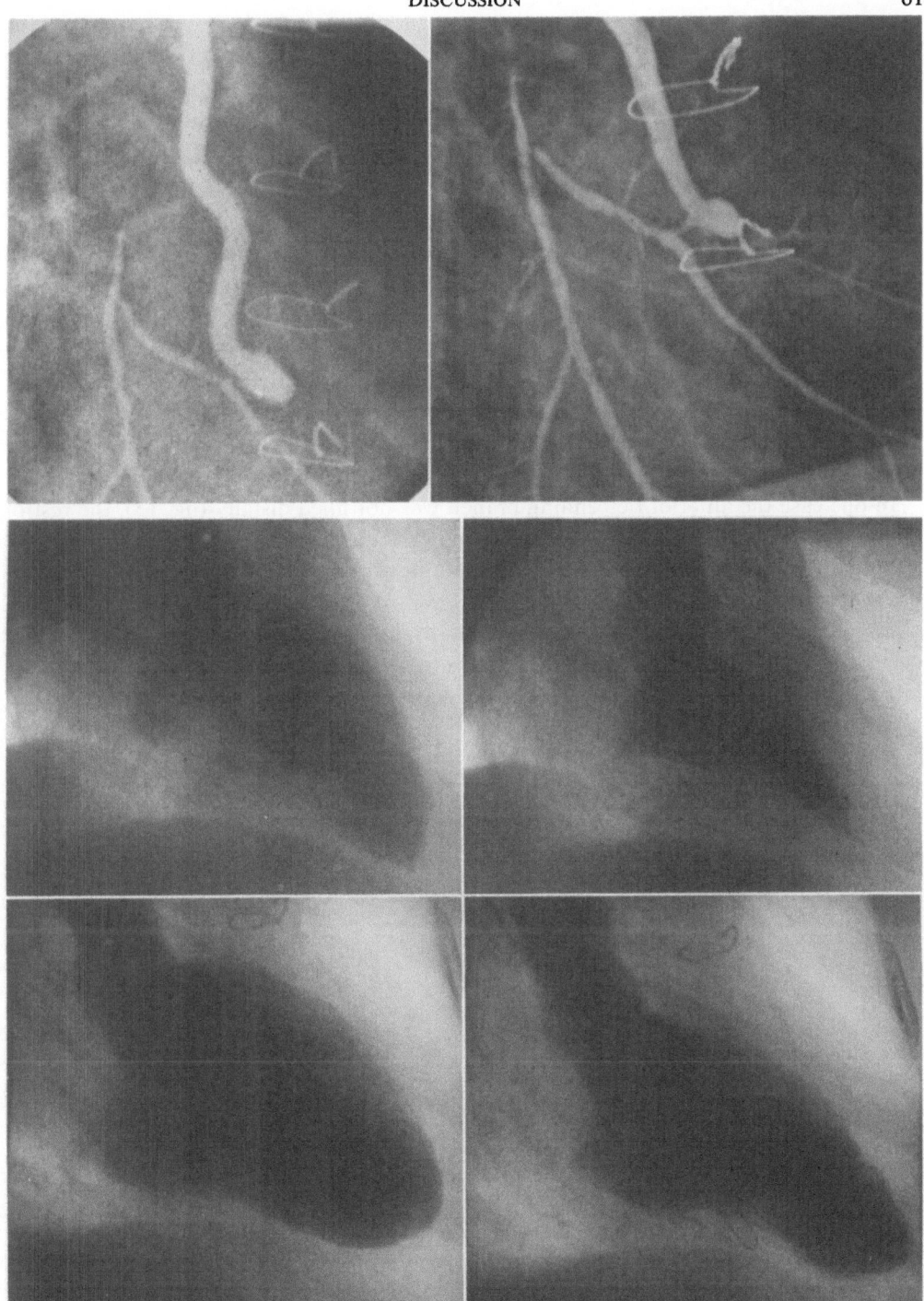

In twenty-one of thirty-eight patients who were re-catheterised one year afterwards, the proximal stenosis in the coronary artery was found to have become total. Figure 35 shows that this can occur as early as two weeks after the operation.

It is striking that if the bypassing vein occludes in the course of time this is rarely reflected in the electrocardiogram, although these patients do appear to have had some symptoms which subsequently justify suspicion of an occlusion.

During the follow-up period three patients sustained a myocardial infarction; in two of them it could be proved that this was related to the occlusion of a vein which was patent immediately after the operation. The time of infarction was eight, thirty and thirty-two months respectively after the operation.

In the first one-hundred patients who were operated on in Leiden a mammary artery was anastomosed with the left coronary artery (anterior descending branch) twelve times, three were occluded directly post-operatively, two were seriously stenosed at the level of the distal anastomosis (figs. 14 and 36).

In one case the anterior descending branch was not filled distally (fig. 15), the rest of the artery being retrogradely filled from the right coronary artery.

The internal mammary artery should have a flow of at least 80 ml/min., if successful use is to be made of it (Flemma et al., 1974).

Endarterectomy was performed only in the right coronary artery and then on eight occasions altogether. The electrocardiograms in two of these eight patients showed an infarct pattern – post-operatively – but the left ventricular angiogram was normal in

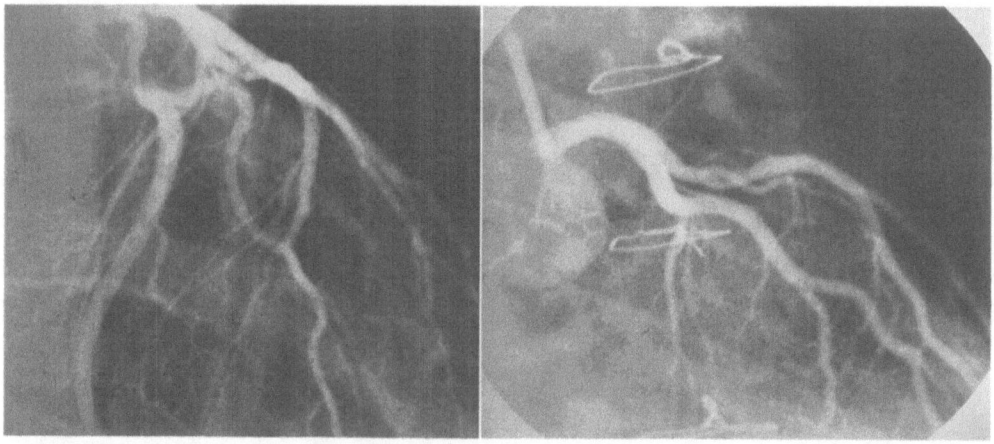

Fig. 35. Left coronary artery in right anterior oblique projection.
Left: before operation with a-stenosis in the left circumflex branch.
Right: after operation subtotal stenosis in left circumflex is now total, due to a vene graft to the circumflex branch (2 weeks post-operative).

both cases. Of these eight patients one died immediately after the operation, in another the graft was occluded. In six the grafts were patent directly post-operatively and in three who were re-catheterised after one year the three grafts were found to be patent.

For the time being endarterectomy seems nevertheless to be a good method for making the distal anastomosis if the lumen of the coronary artery is too small.

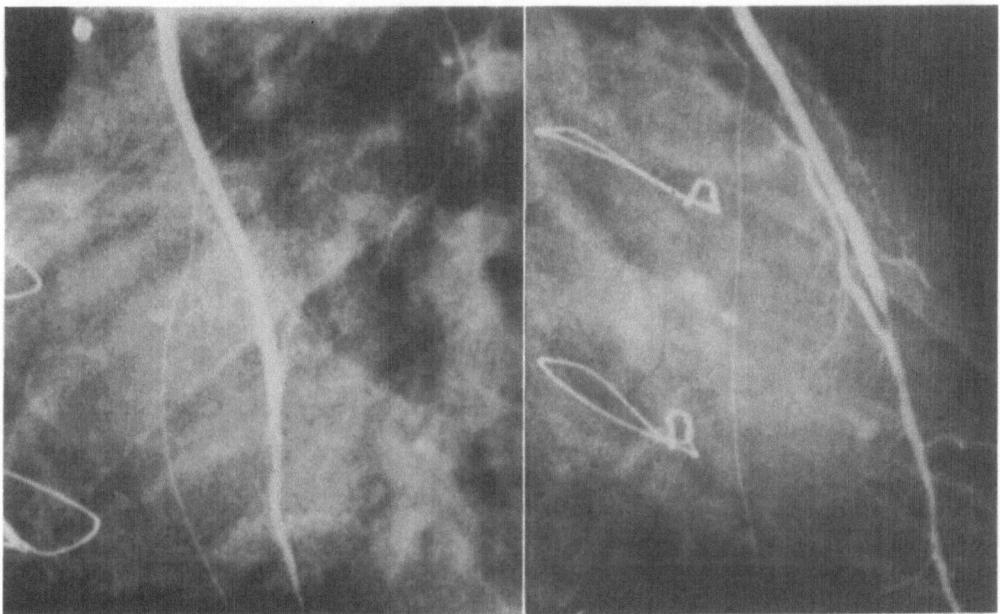

Fig. 36. Left internal mammary artery to the left anterior descending
Left: left anterior oblique projection.
Right: right anterior oblique projection.
Note: severe stenosis just before the distal anastomosis (2 weeks post-operative).

In fifteen of one-hundred and forty-five grafts a stenosis (certainly not present pre-operatively) was seen post-operatively in the bypassed coronary arteries. Figures 15, 16, 37 and 38 show examples of such a stenosis. This abnormality was observed mainly in the anterior descending branch of the left coronary artery. In one single case the bypassing vein sludged in the course of one year. Probably due to a change in the surgical technique this abnormality was observed only once again in a later series of twenty patients, all of whom had been given a graft to the anterior descending branch.

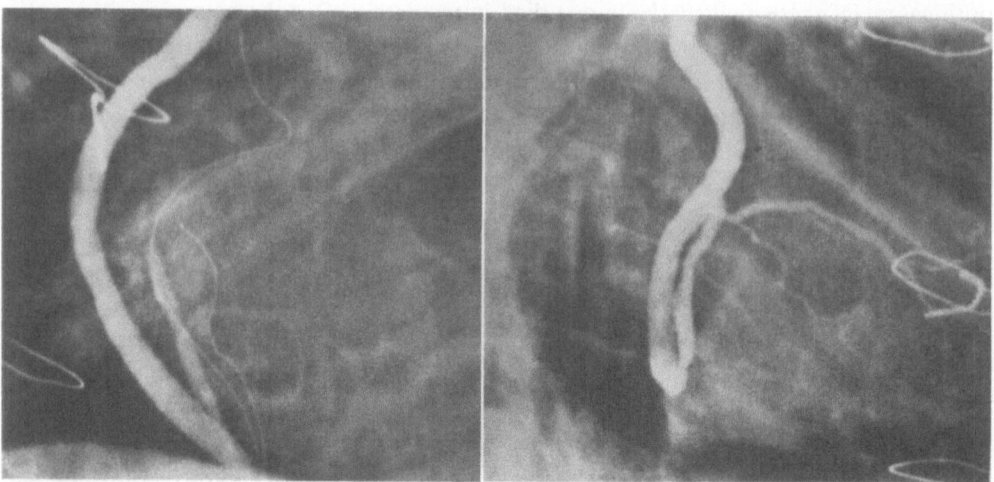

Fig. 37. Saphenous vene graft to the right coronary artery, retrograde filling of the mid part of the artery, complete stenosis of the artery just beyond the distal anastomosis.
Left: left anterior oblique projection.
Right: right anterior oblique projection.

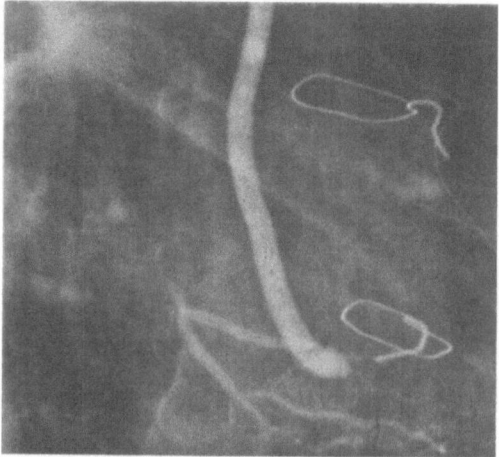

Fig. 38. Saphenous vene graft to the obtuse branch of the left circumflex artery, in right anterior oblique projection, complete stenosis of the artery beyond the distal anastomosis. Directly post-operative.

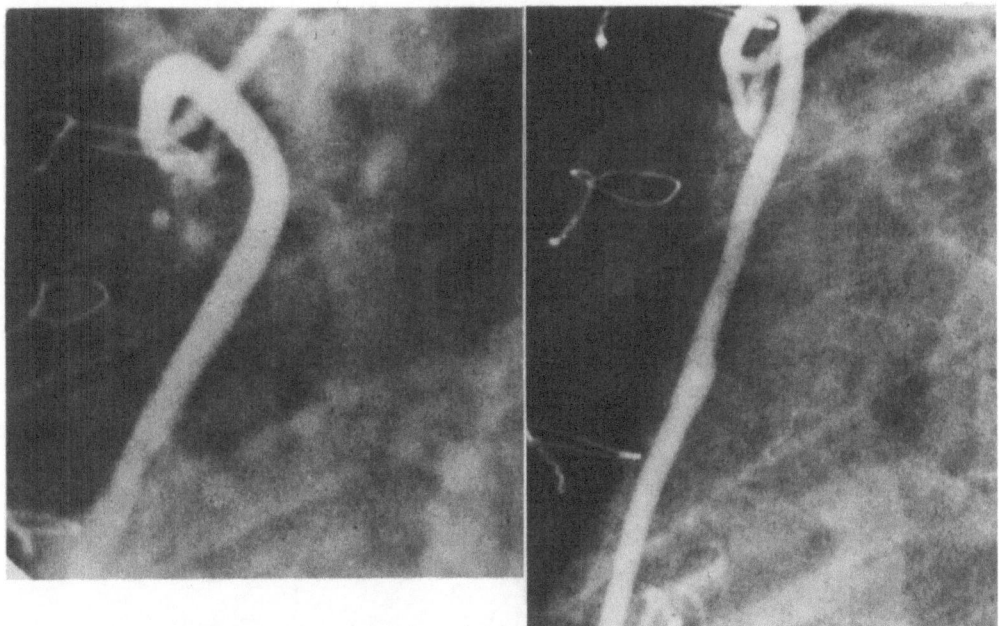

Fig. 39. Saphenous vene graft to the right coronary artery in left anterior oblique projection.
Left: directly post-operative.
Right: one year post-operative.
Note: decrease in diameter of the vene graft. Catheter in both pictures of the same size.

Kaplitt et al. (1971) advocated the use of an X-ray installation in the operating theatre for the purpose of discovering such stenoses during surgery.

We saw this abnormality occur in the right coronary artery and the left circumflex only in 2/58 and 2/10 of cases respectively. Apart from changes in the coronary arteries, a direct post-operative stenosis (figs. 13 and 45) in the bypassing venous grafts was found in 7/145. Just as was the case with the preceding anomaly the cause certainly seemed to lie in the surgical technique.

It was found that abnormalities can also occur in the veins after one year:

1. Reduction in diameter (fig. 39). Bourassa finds that after one year there is no further reduction in diameter. The change in calibre is supposedly caused by the accumulation of acid mucopolysaccharides and fibroblasts in the intima.

2. Local stenosis. A local stenosis not present immediately post-operative was seen one year later in nine of fifty-one grafts (18%). The possibility is not excluded that these abnormalities are the result of damages to the intima of the vein resulting from the operation (figs. 40 and 41). In the case shown in fig. 42 it remains doubtful whether the abnormalities are due to intimal damage. In this patient the stenoses in the proximal coronary artery (not shown here) remain unchanged. It may reasonably be assumed that if this graft occludes altogether, infarction will not occur. It should be considered likely that if such local stenoses can be avoided, the patency rate of the venous bypasses will increase as well.

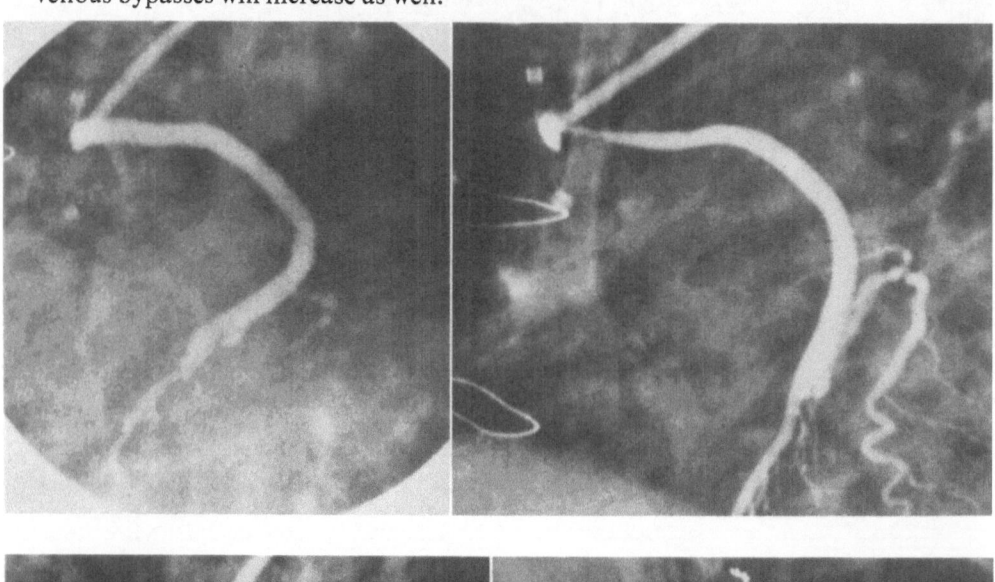

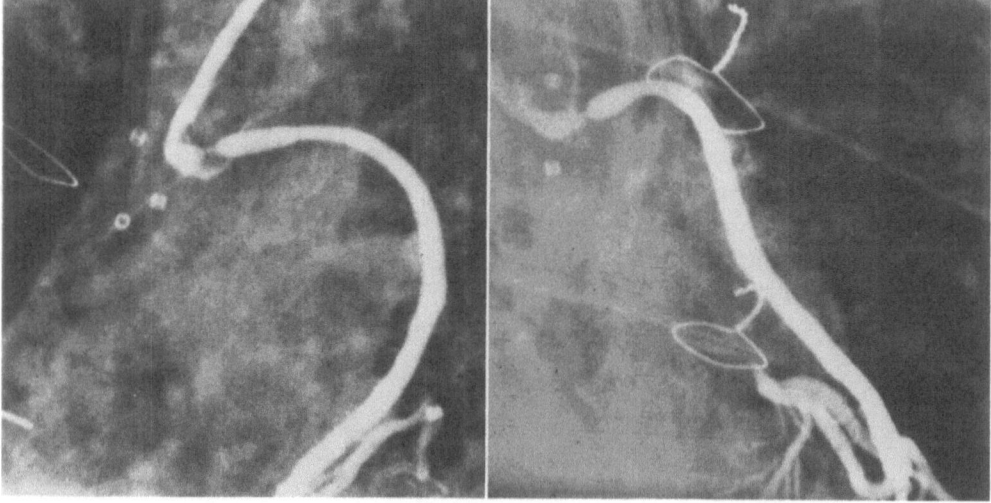

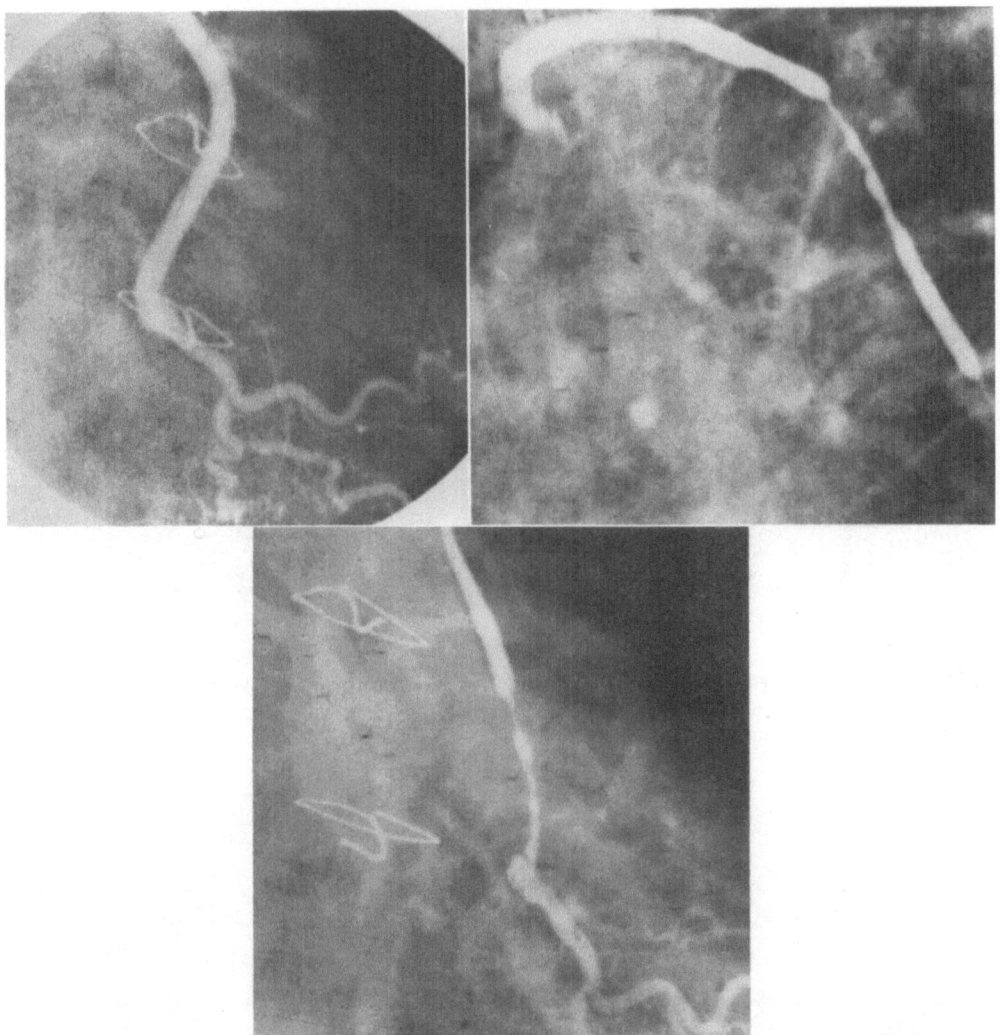

Fig. 42. Saphenous vene graft to the postero-lateral branch of the left circumflex artery.
Top left: directly post-operative.
Top middle: one year post-operative, left anterior oblique projection proximal and mid part of the graft.
Bottom: one year post-operative, right anterior oblique projection, severe narrowing in the distal part.

← *Fig. 40.* Saphenous vene graft to the left anterior descending in left anterior oblique projection.
Left: directly post-operative.
Right: one year post-operative.
Note: severe stenosis in the beginning of the graft after one year.

← *Fig. 41.* Saphenous vene graft to the left anterior descending with a severe stenosis just beyond the proximal anastomosis. One year post-operative.
Left: left anterior oblique projection.
Right: right anterior oblique projection.
Note: directly post-operative normal aspect of the graft.

In the case of gracile coronary arteries as shown in figure 43, the internal mammary artery possibly merits preference to a vein, even though a new implantation of the internal mammary artery in the aorta may be found necessary.

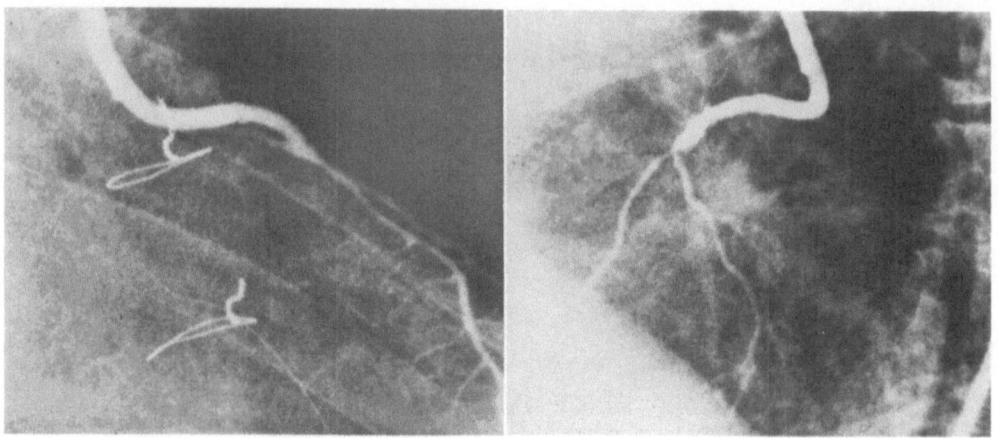

Fig. 43. Saphenous vene graft to small diagonal branch of the left coronary artery. Directly post-operative.
Left: right anterior oblique projection.
Right: left anterior oblique projection.

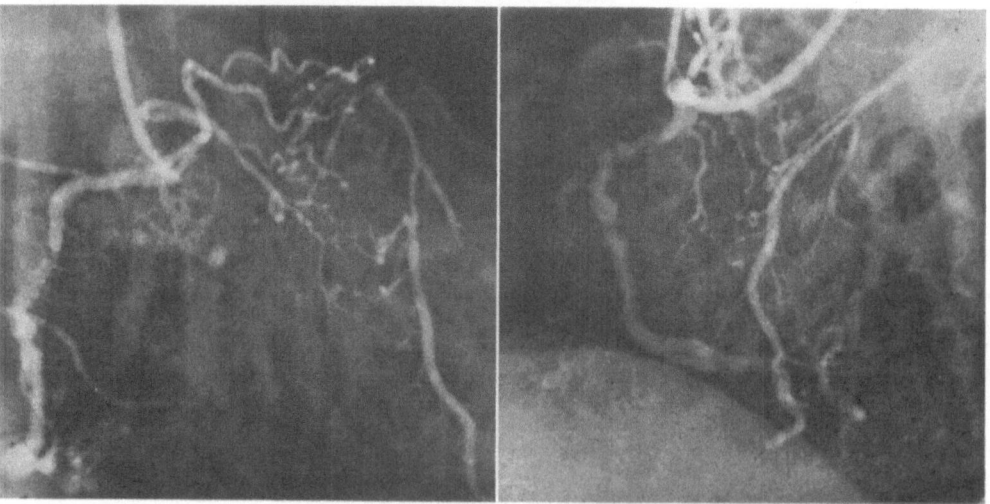

Fig. 44. Collateral filling of the left coronary artery (left anterior descending) by injection in the right coronary artery.
Left: right anterior oblique projection.
Right: left anterior oblique projection.

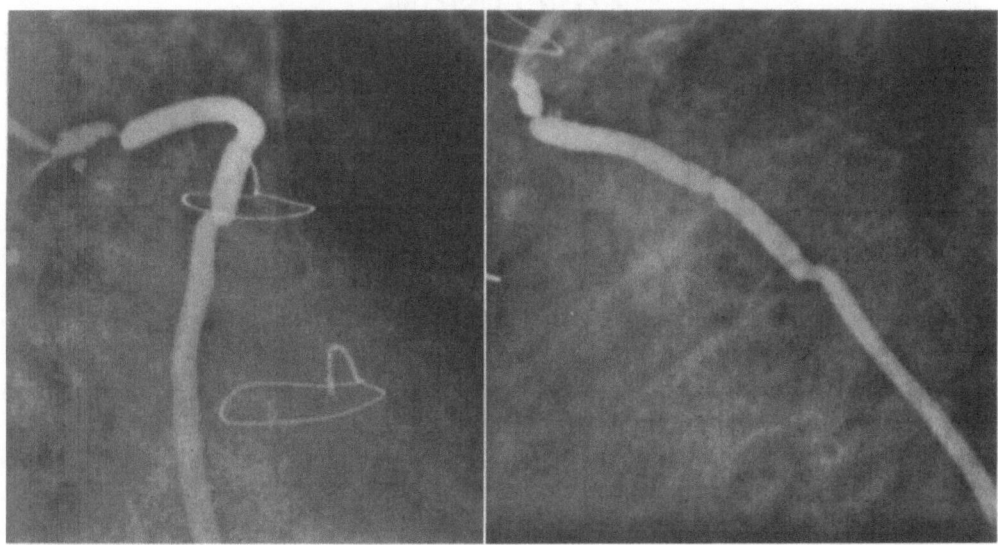

Fig. 45. Saphenous vene graft to the obtuse branch of the left circumflex artery, directly post-operative.
Left: right anterior oblique projection.
Right: left anterior oblique projection.
Note: severe stenosis in the proximal part of the graft. Tip of the catheter wedged in the orifice of the graft.

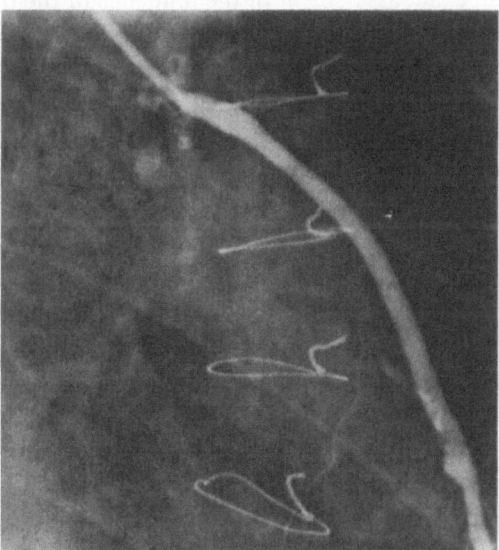

Fig. 46. Saphenous vene graft to the left anterior descending branch of the left coronary artery. 6 months after the operation. Normal aspect of the graft but, the catheter tip always wedged in the orifice of the graft. Aortic angio showed ostium stenosis which was proven by reoperation. Right anterior oblique projection.

CONCLUSIONS

This study reports on findings of clinical and angiographic investigations in 100 patients in whom aorto-coronary bypass surgical procedures were performed. In 12 instances the left internal mammary artery was anastomosed with the anterior descending ramus of the left coronary artery, in the remaining 88 one or more vein grafts were used. In 21 patients it was necessary to carry out other surgical procedures (aneurysmectomy or implantation of an artificial valve) in addition to applying one or more bypasses.

With the evaluation of the data obtained from our series of aorto-coronary bypass operations, we would like to state that:

1. An extensive pre- and post-operative analysis is necessary in order to obtain a proper insight into the surgical treatment of coronary sclerosis.
2. With this extensive analysis it was possible to improve upon not only the indications for operation, but also to provide the surgeon with advice as regards the surgical aspects involved.
3. In order to obtain an exact assessment of the influence of the bypass operation on the patients' life expectancy and risk of (re)myocardial infarction, random testing is necessary.
4. Patients in validity class IV should be excluded from randomization.

REFERENCES

Adam, M., Mitchell, B. F., Lambert, G. J. (1970), Immediate revascularization of the heart. *Circulation* 41, II-73.

Aldridge, H. E., Trimble, A. S. (1971), Progression of proximal coronary artery lesions to total occlusion after aorto-coronary saphenous vein bypass grafting. *J. thorac. cardiovasc. Surg.* 62, 7.

Baddeley, R. M., Ashton, F., Slaney, G., Barnes, A. D. (1970), Late results of autogenous vein bypass grafts in femoropopliteal arterial occlusion. *Brit. med. J.* I, 653.

Bartel, A. G., Behar, V. S., Peter, R. H., Orgain, E. S., King, Y. (1972), Effects of aorto-coronary bypass surgery on treadmill exercise. *Circulation* 46, II-91.

Beck, C. S. (1935), The development of a new bloodsupply to the heart by operation. *Ann. Surg.* 102, 801.

Benchimol, A., Promisloff, S. D., Desser, K. B. (1972), Electrovectorcardiographic changes after proximal right coronary artery venous bypass grafts and distal gas endarterectomy. *Amer. J. Cardiol.* 30, 466.

Blumgart, H. L., Schlesinger, M. J., Davis, D. (1940), Studies on the relation of the clinical manifestations of angina pectoris, coronary thrombosis and myocardial infarction to the pathologic findings with particular reference to the significance of the collateral circulation. *Amer. Heart J.* 19, 1.

Bourassa, M. G., Lespérance, J., Grondin, C. M., Campeau, L. (1971), Factors influencing patency of aorto-coronary vein grafts. *Circulation* 44, II-107.

Bourassa, M. G., Lespérance, J., Campeau, L., Saltiel, J. (1972), Fate of left ventricular contraction following aorto-coronary venous grafts. *Circulation* 46, 724.

Bourassa, M. G., Lespérance, J., Goulet, C., (1972), Progression of coronary arterial disease after aorto-coronary bypass grafts. *Circulation* 46, II-51.

Bruschke, A. V., Proudfitt, W. L., Mason Sones, F. (1973), Progress study of 590 consecutive nonsurgical cases of coronary disease followed 5-9 years. *Circulation* 47, 1147.

Caldwell, R. L., DeWeese, J. A., Rob, C. G. (1968), Femoropopliteal bypass grafts utilizing autogenous veins. *Circulation* 37, 38, II-37.

Campeau, L., Alonzo, F., Elias, G., Bourassa, M. G. (1971), Left ventricular performance during exercise before and after aorto-coronary vein graft surgery. *Circulation* 43, 44, II-148.

Chalmers, T. C. (1972), Randomization and coronary artery surgery. *Ann. thorac. Surg.* 14, 323.

Cohen, M. V., Cohn, P. F., Herman, M. V., Gorlin, R. (1971), Diagnosis and prognosis of main left coronary artery obstruction. *Circulation* 43, 44, II-102.

Cooley, D. A., Hallman, G. L., Wukasch, D. C., Garcia, E., Dawson, J. T., Hall, R. J. (1972), Coronary artery bypass. *Circulation* 45, 46, II-110.

Danielson, G. K., Gau, G. T., Davis, G. D. (1971), Early results of vein bypass grafts for coronary artery disease. *Circulation* 34, 44, II-101.

Darling, R. C., Linton, R. R., Ruzzuk, M. A. (1967), Saphenous vein bypass grafts for femoropopliteal occlusive disease: A reappraisal. *Surgery* 61, 31.

Dart, C. H., Scott, S., Fish, R., Takaro, T. (1970), Direct bloodflow studies of clinical internal thoracic mammary arterial implants. *Circulation* 41, II-64.

Dimond, E. G., Kittle, C. F., Crocket, J. E. (1960), Comparison of internal mammary artery ligation and sham operation for angina pectoris. *Amer. J. Cardiol.* 5, 483.

Dorcahk, J. R., Tristani, F. E., Chaing, L. C., Yoker, J. A. (1971), Left ventricular performance following saphenous vein bypass surgery. *Circulation* 44, II-159.

Edwards, W. S., Blakeley, W. R., Lewis, C. E., Abrams, J. (1972), Coronary bypass entirely with arteries. *Circulation* 45, 46, II-51.

Effler, D. B., (1971), Myocardial revascularization – direct or indirect? *J. thorac. cardiovasc. Surg.* 61, 498.

Effler, D. B., Favaloro, R. G., Groves, L. K., Loop, F. D. (1971), The simple approach to direct coronary artery surgery. *J. thorac. cardiovasc. Surg.* 62, 503.

Effler, D. B., Mason Sones, F., Favaloro, R. G. (1964), Endarterectomy in the treatment of coronary artery disease. *J. thorac. cardiovasc. Surg.* 47, 98.

Effler, D. B., Mason Sones, F., Favaloro, R. G., Groves, L. K. (1965), Coronary endarterectomy with patch graft. *Ann. Surg.* 162, 590.

Effler, D. B., Mason Sones, F., Groves, L. K., Suarez, E. (1965), Myocardial revascularization by Vineberg's internal mammary artery implant. Evaluation of postoperative results. *J. thorac. cardiovasc. Surg.* 50, 527.

Favaloro, R. G. (1967), Saphenous vein autograft replacement of severe segmental coronary artery occlusion. *Ann. thorac. Surg.* 5, 334.

Favaloro, R. G. (1969), Saphenous vein graft in the surgical treatment of coronary artery disease. *J. thorac. cardiovasc. Surg.* 58, 178.

Favaloro, R. G. (1971), Surgical treatment of coronary arteriosclerosis by the saphenous vein graft technique. *J. thorac. cardiovasc. Surg.* 28, 493.

Favaloro, R. G., Effler, D. B., Cheanvechai, C., Quint, R. A., Mason Sones, F. (1971), Acute coronary insufficiency (impending myocardial infarction and myocardial infarction). *Amer. J. Cardiol.* 28, 599.

Favaloro, R. G., Effler, D. B., Groves, L. K., Fergusson, J. G., Lozada, J. S. (1968), Double internal mammary artery-myocardial implantation clinical evaluation of results in 150 patients. *Circulation* 38, 549.

Favaloro, R. G., Effler, D. B., Groves, L. K., Sheldon, W. C., Shirey, E. K., Mason Sones, F. (1970), Severe segmental obstruction of the left main coronary artery and its divisions. *J. thorac. cardiovasc. Surg.* 60, 469.

Flemma, R. J., Singh, H., Tector, A. J., Walker, J. A., Lepley, D. (1974), *Mammary or veingraft in the surgical management of angina pectoris.* Presented at the conference on coronary artery medicine and surgery, Houston, Texas, 1974.

François Frank, C. A. (1899), Signification physiologique de la résection du sympathique dans la maladie de Basedow, l'epilepsie, l'idiotie et le glaucome. *Bull. Acad. nat. Méd.* (Paris) 41, 565.

Friedberg, D. K. (1972), Editorials caution and coronary artery surgery. Timeo chirurgos et dona ferentes. *Circulation* 45, 757.

Friedberg, C. K. (1972), Some comments and reflections in changing interests and new developments in angina pectoris. *Circulation* 46, 1037.

Furuse, A., Klopp, E. H., Brawley, R. K., Gott, V. L. (1972), Hemodynamics of aorta-to-coronary artery bypass. *Ann. thorac. Surg.* 14, 282.

Green, G. E. (1972), Internal mammary artery-to-coronary artery anastomosis. *Ann. thorac. Surg.* 14, 260.

Green, G. E., Spencer, F. C., Tice, D. A., Stertzer, S. H. (1970), Arterial and venous microsurgical bypass grafts for coronary artery disease. *J. thorac. cardiovasc. Surg.* 60, 491.

Green, G. E., Stertzer, S. H., Gordon, R. B., Tice D. A. (1970), Anastomosis of the internal mammary artery to the distal left anterior descending coronary artery. *Circulation* 41, 42, II-79.

Greenberg, B. H., Frahm, C. J., Padilla, D., Giragos, H. G., Hadidian, H. A., Dumanian, A. V. (1971), Arteriographic findings in patients with aorto-coronary saphenous vein bypass grafts and associated manual core endarterectomy. *Circulation* 34, 44, II-102.

Hultgren, H. N., Miyagawa, M., Buck, W., Angell, W. W. (1971), Ischemic myocardial injury during coronary artery surgery. *Amer. Heart J.* 82, 624.

James, T. N. (1961), *Anatomy of the coronary arteries.* Paul B. Hoeber, Inc., New York.

Johnson, W. D., Flemma, R. J., Lepley, D. (1969), Extended treatment of severe coronary artery disease. *Ann. Surg.* 170, 460.

Johnson, W. D., Flemma, R. J., Manley, J. C., Lepley, D. (1970), The physiologic parameters of ventricular function as affected by direct coronary surgery. *J. thorac. cardiovasc. Surg.* 60, 483.

Johnson, W. D., Auer, J. E., Tector, A. J. (1970), Late changes in coronary vein grafts. *Amer. J. Cardiol.* 26, 640.

Johnson, W. D., Lepley, D. (1970), An aggressive surgical approach to coronary disease. *J. thorac. Cardiovasc. Surg.* 59, 128.

Jonnesco, T. (1920), Traitement chirurgical de l'angine de poitrine par la résection du sympathique cervicothoracique. *Bull. Acad. nat. Méd.* (Paris) 84, 93.

Judkins, M. P. (1968), Percutaneous transfemoral selective coronary arteriography. *Radiol. clin. N. Amer.* 6, 467.

Kaplitt, M. J., Robinson, G. (1971), Coronary gas endarterectomy. *Amer. Heart J.* 81, 136.

Kline, S., Apstein, C., Baltaxe, H., Levin, D. (1972), Left ventricular function after aorto-coronary bypass. *Circulation* 45, 46, II-23.

Kolessov, VI. (1967), Mammary artery-coronary artery anastomosis as a method of treatment of angina pectoris. *J. thorac. cardiovasc. Surg.* 54, 535.

Kong, Y., Bartel, A. G., Behar, V. S., Peter, R. H., Morris, J. J., Young, W. G., Oldham, H. N. (1971), Aorto-coronary bypass graft: preoperative correlates of mortality. *Circulation* 43, 44, II-101.

Langston, M. F., Kerth, W. J., Selzer, A., Cohn, K. E. (1972), Evaluation of internal mammary artery implantation. *Amer. J. Cardiol.* 29, 788.

Lichtlen, P. R., Moccetti, T. (1972), Prognostic aspects of coronary angiography. *Circulation* 45, 46, II-7.

Mac Raven, D., Walker, J. A., Friedberg, D., Johnson, W. D. (1972), Survival experience in saphenous vein bypass graft surgery. *Amer. J. Cardiol.* 29, 277.

Manley, J. C., Johnson, W. D., Flemma, R. J., Lepley, D. (1970), Objective evaluation of the effects of direct myocardial revascularization in ventricular performance utilizing submaximal ergometer exercise testing. *Amer. J. Cardiol.* 26, 648.

Mason Sones, F. (1959), *Cine coronary angiography*. Discussion at the second annual symposium cine-fluorography, Rochester N.Y., November 1959.

Mason Sones, F., Shirey, E. K., Proudfitt, W. L., Westcott, R. N. (1959), Cine coronary arteriography. *Circulation* 20, 773.

Mark v. d., F., Frank, H. L. L., Buis, B., Brom, A. G., Bos, E., Nauta, J. (1972), Significance of blood flow measurements in implanted aorta-coronary bypass grafts. *Circulation* 45, 46, II-232.

Matlos, H. J., Alderman, E. L., Wexler, L., Shunway, N. E., Harrison, D. C. (1972), What is the relationship between clinical angina response to coronary surgery and anatomic success? *Circulation* 45, 46, II-50.

May, A. M., Bailey, C. P., Beal, A., Vacco, R. (1969), Operation for coronary artery disease report of the committee in cardiovascular surgery. *Ann. of Chest Physicians: Dis. Chest* 55, 332.

Miller, S. E. P., Johnson, W. D., Tector, A. J., Manley, J. C., Gale, H. H. (1972), The effect of myocardial revascularization on anginal symptoms, ventricular function and exercise performance. *Circulation* 45, 46, II-24.

Moberg, C. H., Webster, J. S., Mason Sones, F. Jr. (1972), Natural history of severe proximal coronary disease as defined by angiography. *Amer. J. Cardiol.* 29, 282.

Morris, G. C., Reul, G. J., Howell, J. F., Crawford, E. S., Chapman, D. W., Beazley, H. L., Winters, W. L., Peterson, P. K., Lewis, J. M. (1972), Follow up results of distal coronary artery bypass for ischemic heart disease. *Amer. J. Cardiol.* 29, 180.

Murray, G., Porcheron, R., Hilario, J. E., Roschlauw, (1954), Anostomosis of a systemic artery to the coronary. *Canad. med. Ass. J.* 71, 594.

Reul, G. J., Morris, G. C., Howell, J. F., Crawford, E. S., Sandiford, F. M., Wukasch D. C. (1971), The safety of ischemic cardiac arrest in distal coronary artery bypass. *J. thorac. cardiovasc. Surg.* 62, 511.

Reul, G. J., Morris, G. C., Howell, J. F., Crawford, E. S., Stelter, W. J. (1972), Current concepts in coronary artery surgery. *Ann. thorac. Surg.* 14, 243.

Senning, A. (1961), Strip grafting in coronary arteries. *J. thorac. cardiovasc. Surg.* 41, 542.

Sheldon, W. C., Rincon, G., Effler, D. B., Proudfitt, W. L., Mason Sones, F. (1972), Vein graft surgery for coronary artery disease: Survival and angiographic results among the first one thousand patients. *Circulation* 45, 46, II-110.

Spodick, D. H. (1971), Revascularization of the heart, numerators in search of denominators. *Amer. Heart J.* 81, 149.

Taylor, W. J., Gorlin, R. (1967), Objective criterial for internal mammary artery implantation. *Ann. thorac. Surg.* 4, 143.

Thompson, S. A., Raisbeek, M. I. (1949), Surgical rehabilitation of coronary cripple. *Ann. internal Med.* 31, 1010.

Vineberg, A. M. (1962), Surgery of coronary artery disease. *Progr. cardiovasc. Dis.* 4, 391.

Vlodaver, Z., Edwards, J. E. (1971), Pathologic changes in aortic coronary arterial saphenous vein grafts. *Circulation* 44, 719.

Walker, J. A., Friedberg, H. D., Flemma, R. J., Johnson, W. D. (1971), Determinants of angiographic patency of aorto-coronary vein bypass grafts. *Circulation* 34, 44, II-108.

Walker, J. A., Friedberg, H. D., Flemma, R. J., Johnson, W. D. (1972), Determinants of angiographic patency of aorto-coronary vein bypass grafts. *Circulation* 45, I-86.

Yatteau, R. F., Peter, R. H., Bartel, A. G., Behar, V. S., Kong, Y. (1972), Ischemic myocardiopathy. *Circulation* 45, 46, II-24.

X-RAY CATHETERISATION SYSTEM

An X-ray catheterisation installation or system consists of a number of elements. Most of the characteristics of the total system are determined by the related characteristics of several components. The choice of the components, moreover, has been determined also by their mutual compatibility and their possibilities within the system.

A description of the separate components will be followed by a consideration of the parameters to be adjusted, and of the over-all characteristics of the system in use. The arrangement of the components is reproduced schematically in the figure on page 00. (The system as described was supplied by Philips Medical Systems Division and has been in use since the end of 1972.)

The high-tension generator, type MAXIMUS 100, has a 12-valve rectifying circuit and a thyristor-controlled time switch. By means of the latter, switching times with short durations (down to 1 ms) are possible up to a frequency of 12 per second. The maximum tension available from the generator is 150 kV, and the highest power 100 kW.

A Cine-Pulse unit is incorporated in the circuit to the X-ray tube. With this unit, equally short switching times (minimal 1 ms) can be obtained up to a frequency of 400 per second. The use of the Cine-Pulse unit limits the X-ray tube current to 300 mA.

The X-ray tube is of the Super ROTALIX type. Two versions have been used, one with a 0.6 and 1.2 mm focus, and another with a 0.6 and 1.5 mm focus. The maximal tube load amounts to 20/50 kW and 30/100 kW respectively. The dimensions of the X-ray beam are adjusted by a remote-controlled collimator.

The circular grid in front of the 6 inch image intensifier has 24 lines per cm, a ratio of 7, and a focus distance of 85 cm. The 6 inch image intensifier has a caesium iodide primary screen. The diameter of the secondary screen is 16.8 mm.

With the optical attachment, the image on the secondary screen of the image intensifier can be distributed in different directions. The three-channel optical attachment shown here is connected to a TV-camera, a rapid-sequence camera and a cine-camera. Furthermore it is possible to direct the optical image in two directions simultaneously. Thus, during a cinefluorographic or rapid-sequence camera recording, it is possible to follow the process instantly on the TV-monitor. The image distributor contains a basic lens of 0.85/58 mm.

A photomultiplier tube is incorporated in the optical attachment to measure the light emitted by a part of the secondary screen of the image intensifier. When a certain value is reached, the radiation can be switched off either via the generator itself (thyristor controlled time switch), or via the Cine-Pulse unit.

The Arriflex camera (35 mm) can operate at up to 80 frames per second. The images are over-framed by the use of a 2.0/85 mm camera lens. The image frame is 18 × 24 mm. The camera initiates the radiation pulse by means of a signal to the Cine-Pulse unit.

The rapid-sequence camera has an image size of 70 mm, and a frequency up to 6 frames per second. The images are over-framed by the use of a 5.1/300 mm lens. Exposure release is initiated by a pulse coming directly from the camera to the generator.

The TV-system comprises a camera with a Plumbicon tube, a stabilising circuit and a monitor. The stabilising circuit controls the X-ray intensity via the generator in such a way that for a certain part of the image, the signal current from the TV-camera does not exceed a specified limit. The TV-monitor has a 19 inch screen. Fluoroscopy is switched by foot. The TV-images may be recorded by a video-recorder.

The patient lies in a cradle which is mounted on an Angio DIAGNOST stand. The working-height can be varied by motor drive between 85 and 110 cm from the floor. The cradle can be rotated around its longitudinal axis to 70° in one direction, and 110° in the other. Moreover, the cradle may be shifted in longitudinal and transverse directions over distances of 90 cm and 25 cm respectively. (The cradle can easily be exchanged for a flat table top.) As the table support is located at one end of the stand, equipment can be moved under the table in the longitudinal direction. An under-table tube is mounted in a carriage coupled to a carriage-mounted film changer. The height of the tube in the carriage can be adjusted. After fluoroscopic positioning using the under-table tube, a film changer series can thus be made with the over-table tube without moving the patient. The movements of cradle and stand and the collimator can be controlled by the physician during catheterisation.

The total system is earthed centrally in the support column. All electric leads go via a panel in the support column, and are connected by means of plugs.

The physiological data required are obtained with the aid of Statham pressure transducers and a Philips eight-channel ultraviolet recorder. The derivatives of the ECG and pressures are reproduced simultaneously on two monitors connected in parallel, one located in the examination room, and the other in the control room.

When using contrast medium containing iodine, as in angiography, the images have more contrast at lower X-ray energies, i.e. at lower tube tensions.

The ideal is a tension of around 70 kV. Another parameter affecting the image quality is the exposure time. It is known from practice that in coronary examinations an exposure time of less than 3 ms causes no perceptable movement blur, and that the blurring caused by an exposure time of 5 ms is still acceptable. On the other hand, the capacity of the X-ray tube and, when applicable, the Cine-Pulse unit has to be taken into account.

The closeness with which the target values given above can be approached depends strongly on the absorption of the object. In practice, with an increasing absorption one initially prolongs the exposure time from 3 up to 5 ms, then the larger focus of the X-ray tube is chosen. If the density is still insufficient, the tube tension is increased. With the system described here, the tube tension does not have to exceed 100 kV. By way of exception, with very thick patients, the X-ray tube may be raised to reduce the distance to patient and image intensifier by 25 cm. (The usual distance between X-ray tube and image intensifier is 90 to 100 cm.) A disadvantage of this reduction is the fact that only a smaller part of the object is recorded on one image.

When making test exposures, the most absorbent parts of the object to be recorded should be positioned in the centre of the beam. If a large quantity of contrast medium is expected in the centre of the beam, the exposure control can be switched off by means of a 'lock-in' circuit, and the original tube current will remain constant.

Cinefluorography is the method of choice for recording rapidly occurring phenomena. In general, an exposure frequency of 50 frames per second is used. This has the additional advantage that there is then no interference with the TV-image. Usually, ten 7-second series are made per examination.

A rapid-sequence camera is used to record single images for closer study. For a good quality image, a single exposure will require about four times the entrance dose needed for a single cine frame. A rapid-sequence series usually consists of about fifteen images made at a rate of two per second, and an average of four series are made per examination. An advantage is that the films can be rapidly processed, and given an initial inspection during the examination.

Use of the full-size film changer is indicated in the rarely occurring event of the size of the object exceeding the format of the input screen of the image intensifier, e.g. in studies of the pulmonary vessels.

The average duration of fluoroscopy per examination is around 14 minutes, and calculations show that the average dose during fluoroscopy is somewhat less than that required for cinefluoroscopy. The dose required for the rapid-sequence exposures per examination is usually less than one-tenth of that required for cinefluorography.

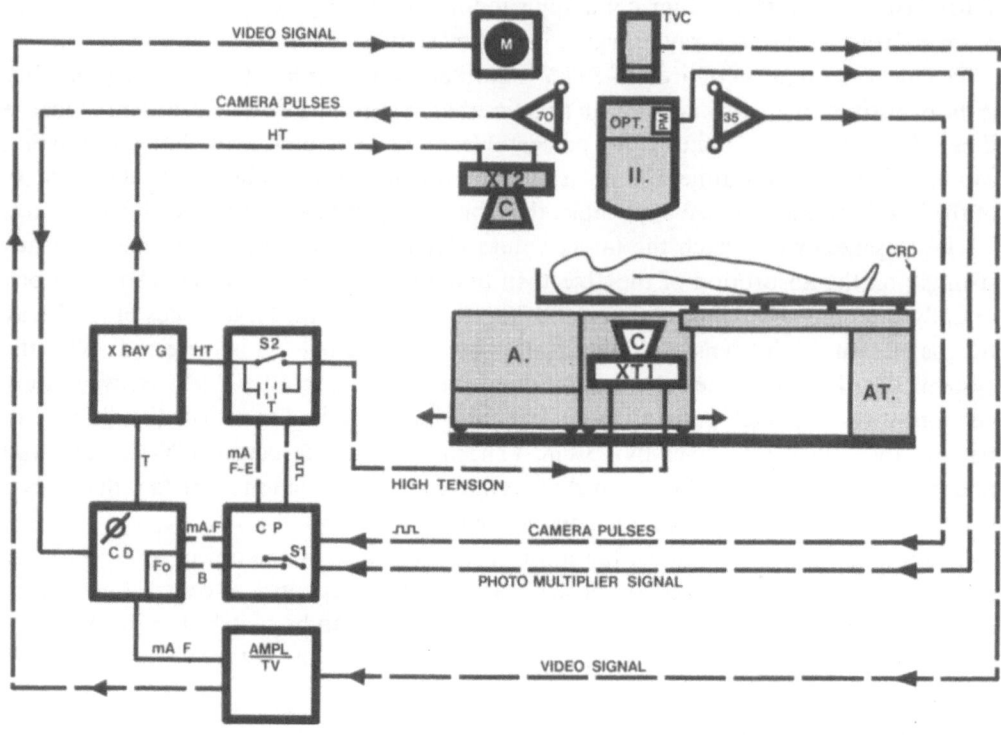

M	– monitor	Fo	– phototimer for 70 mm photo-camera	
TVC	– T.V. camera			
70	– 70 mm photo-camera	X-RAY G	– X-ray generator	
35	– 35 mm cine-camera	T	– Cine-Pulse-tetrode tank	
OPT	– three-channel optical attachment	XT2	– X-ray tube for rapid film changer	
PM	– photomultiplier	S1	– photomultiplier signal for cine or rapid-sequence camera	
II	– image intensifier			
CRD	– cradle	S2	– high-tension switch for cine or for rapid-sequence camera (switch closed)	
AT	– angio-table			
C	– collimator			
A	– rapid film changer	HT	– high tension	
XT1	– X-ray tube for image intensifier	T	– low tension	
TV AMP	– T.V. amplifier	mA F	– mA control for fluoroscopy	
CP	– Cine-Pulse unit	mA F-E	– mA control for fluoroscopy and exposure	
CD	– control desk			

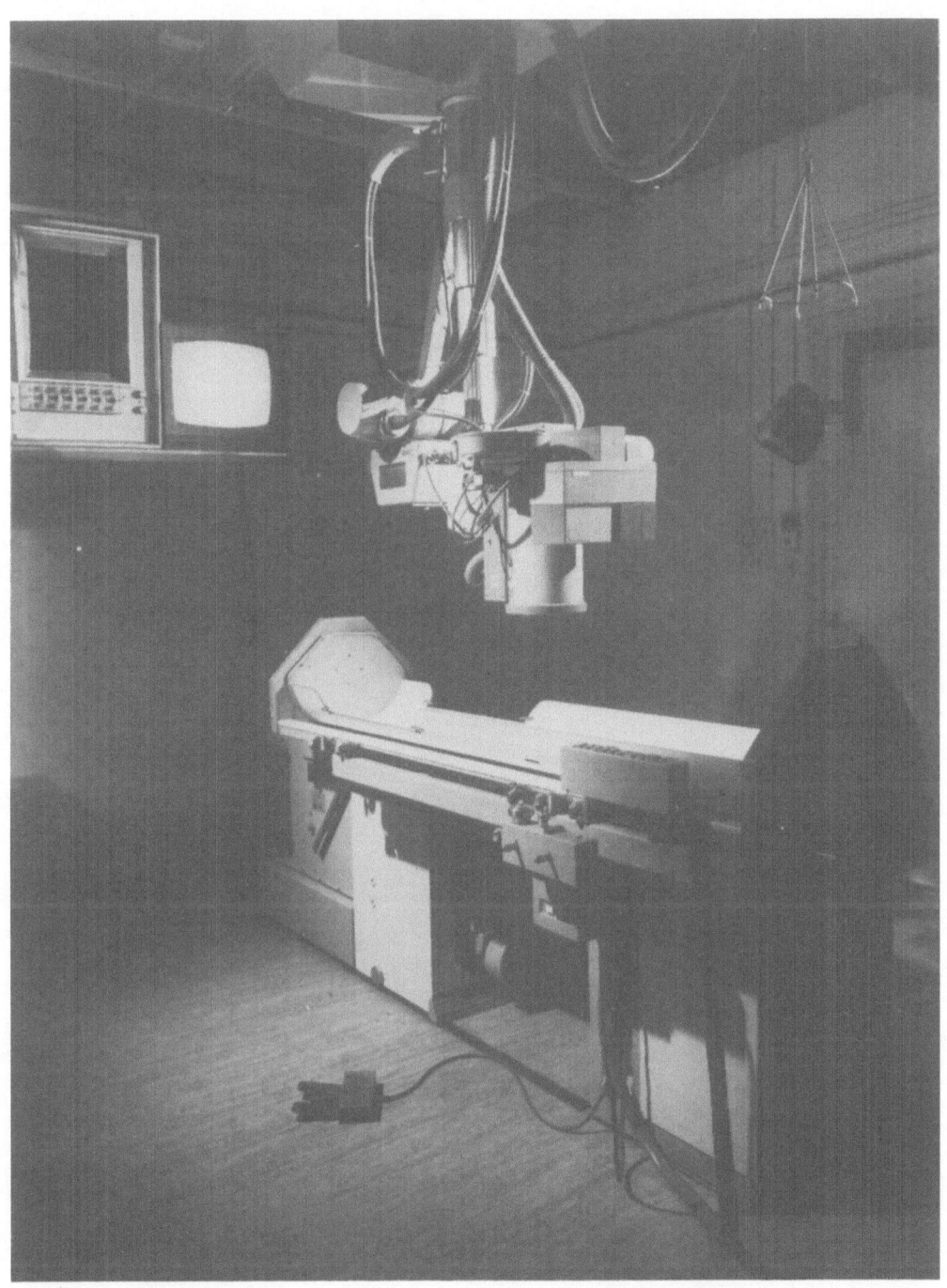